Rx *for*
Survival

The Penguin Press
New York
2005

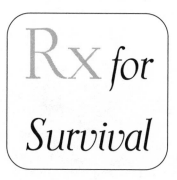

Rx *for* Survival

WHY WE

MUST RISE TO THE

GLOBAL HEALTH

CHALLENGE

PHILIP J. HILTS

THE PENGUIN PRESS

Published by the Penguin Group

Penguin Group (USA) Inc., 375 Hudson Street, New York, New York 10014, U.S.A. •
Penguin Group (Canada), 90 Eglinton Avenue East, Suite 700, Toronto, Ontario, Canada M4P 2Y3
(a division of Pearson Penguin Canada Inc.) • Penguin Books Ltd, 80 Strand, London WC2R ORL,
England • Penguin Ireland, 25 St. Stephen's Green, Dublin 2, Ireland (a division of Penguin
Books, Ltd) • Penguin Books Australia Ltd, 250 Camberwell Road, Camberwell, Victoria 3124,
Australia (a division of Pearson Australia Group Pty Ltd) • Penguin Books India Pvt Ltd,
11 Community Center, Panchsheel Park, New Delhi–110 017, India • Penguin Group (NZ),
Cnr Airborne and Rosedale Roads, Albany, Auckland 1310, New Zealand (a division of Pearson
New Zealand Ltd) • Penguin Books (South Africa) (Pty) Ltd, 24 Sturdee Avenue,
Rosebank, Johannesburg 2196, South Africa

Penguin Books Ltd, Registered Offices:
80 Strand, London WC2R ORL, England

First published in 2005 by the Penguin Press, a member of Penguin Group (USA) Inc.

ISBN 1-59420-070-X

Printed in the United States of America

1   3   5   7   9   10   8   6   4   2

Designed by Claire Vaccaro

To Carisa

ACKNOWLEDGMENTS

I want to thank Gloria Loomis, agent extraordinaire, and Emily Loose, editor at The Penguin Press who believed in the project and shaped the book under deadline pressure. For help along the way I want to thank Paula Apsell, Larry Klein, Lisa Mirowitz, and Gaia Remerowski, who worked on the Public Television Series *Rx for Survival*; William Wester, Carolyn Wester, Michelle Schaan, Debbie Small, Michael Cassell, and Gillian Goodwin in Botswana; Penny Dawson, Steve LeClerq, and Pooja Pandey in Nepal; Fazle Abed and David Sack in Bangladesh; Larry Slutsker, Mary Hamel, and Juliana Otieno in Kenya; and Naysan Sahba and Sudeep Gadok Singh in India.

CONTENTS

Introduction

A Time to Choose

The most pressing issue of our time is not war or the threat of terrorism, serious as those challenges are. Those political conflicts
crowd our field of vision, but there is a deeper, more lasting trend that
will prove more important in the long run. The tide has begun to turn
against us in the fight against deadly diseases and the promotion of
general health and longevity. For the past 150 years humankind has
made historic progress in fighting disease and, much more broadly, in
extending both the length and quality of life around the planet. But
now we face a crucial moment in history, as diseases have begun roar-
ing back. The resurgence in disease in both the rich and poor nations
has consequences not only for our health, but for basic social and political stability all around the world. The rise in health is the base of
human progress, and in a world more globally interconnected than
ever before, we cannot let the many years of progress collapse without
grave consequences in both the developing and the developed nations.

To understand the urgency of the choice we must make now, we must appreciate how dramatically globalization is quickening, and what the vital links are between globalization and world health. After 9/11, some thought that terrorism and war would derail globalization, but, after only a pause, it has accelerated. This global boom actually started during the economic recovery following World War II, but it has picked up speed with the ending of the cold war. The scale is breathtaking. As of the end of 2004 the people of the world spent 250 billion minutes of air time on international calls. We made a billion trips between countries. The size of the global economy has increased 700 percent since 1950. The volume of world trade was sixteen times greater in 2000 than it was in 1950, and it has continued to rise substantially.

Before this boom, there was an earlier one starting in the nineteenth century, shooting up a volcanic plume of economic growth that circled the globe with its effects. It created great riches in England and Europe and propelled the long rise of world capitalism, driven in large part by new technologies. In that phase of rapid change we created the telegraph, telephone, airplane, railway, and automobile, and opened both the Panama and the Suez canals. Communication flourished: By 1890, more than fifty thousand cables had been sent across the Atlantic, and more than a million telephones were operating in the United States alone.

Once again in today's globalization we enjoy an impressive array of new technologies, including jet travel, ever more powerful computers, satellites, the Internet, and cell phones. In 1960 the cost of a three-minute telephone call from New York to London was $60.42; in 1980 it was $6.32; and in 1990 it was just $0.40. In 1996 Internet users numbered 30 million; in 2003 there were 688 million. The links forged in the last globalization now seem like mere rope bridges compared to today's world nerve network.

The payoff of this accelerated globalization could be large, spreading new prosperity especially in rapidly developing countries such as India and China. But we must also be alert: This kind of speed and scale of human interactions creates unexpected hazards. For example, if we count only travel between the nations with a heavy burden of disease and those with less disease, more than a million people a week are making the trip. In that figure we can begin to see the problem: History tells us that along with globalization come both disease and social disruption. The first great globalization is often also called both the "era of epidemics" and the "era of revolution."

It has taken political analysts and economists some time to understand the connection between economic boom and social disruption, but now we know enough to be worried. The new phase of globalization could lead to the creation of not only wealth but suffering on an entirely new scale. As Thomas Friedman of the *New York Times* suggests in *The World Is Flat,* the next time your computer has problems you will be talking to someone in India for instructions on how to fix it, and in Missouri your McDonald's drive-up order will be flashed to someone nine hundred miles away and back. The opportunities in such a highly interconnected world are impressive. Intimate connections, however, can cut both ways. Diseases—as well as goods and services—travel with much greater speed and reach in such a world, as do their human counterparts, terrorists.

The dangers that arise from intense globalization are many, but one of the most fearful is that of disease epidemics. This is the bad news in globalization: The transmission of goods and the transmission of disease are inseparable. Historically, they are not just similar in moving from port to port or airport to airport; they are the same events.

When the black plague made its way to a port on the Black Sea in the 1300s, goods were carried aboard and lice-infested rats came with them for the ride. Both the goods and the disease arrived in Europe on the same ship. In the nineteenth century, when cholera had made its way to the Baltic Sea, a sailor caught the germ and then got on board a lumber boat bound for England. Timber and disease arrived as fellow passengers.

Despite our best efforts the link between trade and disease has persisted. In 1985, a shipment of used tires from Japan arrived in an American port. The tires had small pockets of water inside—where Asian mosquitoes were breeding. These mosquitoes were of the species that transmit the new, more virulent strain of dengue fever. Thus, a scourge of a century ago in the Americas has returned again, hitchhiking its way in truck tires.

The avian flu appears ready to jump from an animal outbreak to a full-scale human-to-human epidemic, and a report of the National Academy of Sciences in the U.S. gave an example of a near miss in which avian flu almost made it to Europe: "Two eagles were smuggled into Belgium from Thailand. Customs officials at Brussels airport found and seized the birds, which were then discovered to be infected with H5N1 and immediately culled . . . and destroyed." It was a close call; avian flu has not yet appeared outside Asia, but it continues to spread there.

People themselves are also excellent vessels of disease transport. When AIDS broke through the surface of human consciousness in 1981 only gradually did biologists and epidemiologists realize what they were looking at when they peered down at this unusual virus. The disease seemed to be an isolated outbreak of a disease organism from some isolated spot in a jungle somewhere. It was a particularly tough case as well, because they knew nothing about its makeup or its behavior. They discovered that it enters the body and then goes silent for many years while the infected human body unwittingly passes it on to others. It later breaks out, not in the form of its own recognizable disease, but with an attack on the whole defense system. All of that was learned within the first few years of the appearance of HIV. What was not clear for some time, however, was that these scientists were looking at a new era in epidemic disease in which more new bacteria viruses and other microbes were appearing in the world than ever before.

So far in this globalization one outbreak of new disease has gone out of control—AIDS, which is taking a staggering economic and social toll in many countries. But those who think we are sure to escape further pandemics of disease, due to our state-of-the-art medical technologies, are those who haven't read biology. Word of outbreaks of disease appears almost daily in newspapers, stories of new diseases gaining more footholds or of old diseases recovering ground. In the spring of 2005 we heard news of the deadly hemorrhagic Marburg fever spreading in Africa, and of the reentry of polio into Indonesia after years of absence.

Just as in the last great globalization, we are in fact seeing today a surge in deadly new diseases and an increased risk of global outbreaks.

A startling number of new diseases have emerged in recent years, including AIDS, mad cow disease, hantavirus, *E. coli,* Lyme, West Nile, SARS, and avian flu. Altogether, forty new diseases—a record as far as we can tell—have appeared since 1973. In addition, twenty diseases that had been suppressed have roared back, including dengue fever, cholera, and tuberculosis. Malaria, eradicated from the Western world and significantly reduced in Africa, has reasserted its presence there, rising again as one of the top killers of children on the continent with more than a million deaths annually. Epidemiologists have noted that outbreaks of food-borne diseases have multiplied fivefold in the past two decades.

This fuller picture of the meaning of AIDS and the threat of other new diseases took form, starting in 1998, as a new wave of disease emerged and was described in a series of reports issued by the Institute of Medicine of the National Academy of Sciences, the most distinguished body of scientists in America. The findings were popularized in a sobering bestselling book, *The Coming Plague,* by immunologist and writer Laurie Garrett, a few years later.

One thing the appearance of AIDS indicated was that our disease surveillance was lax. The disease had existed for fifty years, and in humans for at least twenty years, before we spotted it, by accident, when an unusual number of orders came in for a pneumonia medicine. We might well have diverted the course of the world epidemic if we had not let our public health vigilance drop.

Recognition of the disease threat grew, and when the top experts met in 1992 to review the subject, they reported the news of the emergence of so many new diseases and resurgence of old ones, and high-lighted that we had slipped backward in our monitoring of disease threats and other public health efforts. U.S. government spending on public health reached a peak in 1970, then dropped dramatically to less than half its former level, and remained low through 2000. We forgot that we had to run hard to keep up, and so we began to slip back just as the risk of epidemic outbreaks was escalating.

Tuberculosis offers a telling example of those choices and their consequences. Government health offices had made great progress in combating TB during the twentieth century, and it had been reduced to a steady, low level. In the United States in the 1980s research on TB waned, and in 1986 the TB surveillance program of the Centers for Disease Control was terminated. Then, in 1989, a new proposal was made within the U.S. Department of Health and Human Services to knock down tuberculosis once and for all with a program of reaching out to treat pockets of cases around the United States. This proposal was to make a push to eliminate TB entirely in the United States. But because Congress had cut funds for public health projects, getting this project off the ground proved impossible. As if on cue, surges of the disease started up in many areas in 1989. An additional twenty-eight thousand cases were reported over the next five years.

Adding to the problem is the fact that vaccine development has slowed, with only half the number of companies that are licensed to make them still actually producing them. We are now relying on the vaccines of the 1960s and 1970s, despite our greater knowledge of the basic science.

All of this disease evolution was natural and should have been expected. Bacteria and viruses are automatic duplicating and evolving machines; if you create a drug to kill germs or clean germs out of an environment, the nature of germs is to multiply and change until they can beat the drug or reenter the environment. Victories over troublesome biology are temporary, so vigilance must be constant.

The accelerating globalization is only exacerbating the problem. Travel between nations is three orders of magnitude higher than in the early twentieth century. In addition, the destruction and thus opening of isolated habitats has also increased by orders of magnitude. This combination allows germs to escape their local habitats, travel great distances, and mix with other germs to become more potent.

When forests and other largely untouched locales are leveled and occupied by humans, the germ reservoirs there spill out their organisms. And today, when these microbes reach humans and their animals, they don't stay put. In 1950 there were few large roads traversing Africa; now there is essentially no place left unopened—even the last refuges of the gorilla and the lion are pierced by roads. At the ends of the roads are bus stops, train terminals, and airports.

AIDS followed just such a route. Before AIDS arrived in America it was incubated in apes. The disease probably first made its way to humans by infecting those who lived and worked around apes and who sometimes eat apes as "game meat." From those remote reservoirs in rural Africa it arrived in nearby cities such as Kinshasa, in what is now the Democratic Republic of the Congo. By plane from there the virus arrived in St. Louis, Missouri, and probably other places, including spots in the Caribbean islands.

The increased potency of microbes today comes from gene swapping among them. For example, a virus that infects birds, such as a flu that commonly infects chickens in rural China, may infect the body of a pig on a nearby pig farm. Though the flu may not be able to cause disease in the pig at first, it might pick up new genetic material from the pig, and in the game of Russian roulette that is microbial evolution, that genetically changed form of flu might then be able to infect humans. Just this scenario has been responsible for the appearance of the H5N1 flu virus, an avian flu that has killed millions of birds in Asia and, more recently, fifty-three humans as of the middle of 2005. This is the flu that made its way to Belgium via the two eagles smuggled from Thailand mentioned earlier. Fortunately, the fact that the eagles were infected was discovered quickly and the birds were killed. Scientists fear that a similar episode will one day not be stopped short and the flu will move from continent to continent.

The more viruses and bacteria that meet one another inside the bodies of pigs, birds, and people, the more trading happens. As in roulette, the more spins of the wheel, the greater the chances that a new, virulent form of a disease will emerge.

Historically, the first great outbreak of such newly evolved diseases from their animal reservoirs occurred when humans left their small tribal groups and began to build towns, more than eight thousand years ago. Living in denser populations allowed disease organisms to pass from person to person faster, infecting more people in a shorter time and sustaining an outbreak for a longer time. At the same time humans domesticated a long list of animals, bringing much new microbial baggage into contact with human populations. Scholars note that the story of the Garden of Eden might have arisen during this time, when humans looked back to a period in which rampant disease was not present among human tribes. The contest between microbes and humans eventually reached some stasis. But then we began our intercontinental travels, which resulted in a rush of new outbreaks. At first, the outbreaks were regional, though the regions covered were quite wide.

The Black Death, or bubonic plague, spread from Asia to Europe and killed possibly a third of the population of Europe between 1347 and 1352. Spanish conquistadors brought smallpox to the Americas, where it killed a third to a half of the population of Native Americans who encountered it, thus ensuring the victory of the small number of soldiers over the extended Inca and Aztec empires. Syphilis ran like wildfire in Europe after 1490, possibly brought back from America by explorers. Then came the first truly worldwide epidemic, the cholera waves of 1830 to 1890.

The most deadly and most global single outbreak yet was the famous 1918 influenza epidemic, the "Spanish flu," that emerged in the midwestern area of the United States and spread to every population on earth. During its worst six months it killed 30 million to 40 million people—mostly young, healthy people—and is now counted as the single greatest demographic shock to have occurred in human history. Altogether over three years the flu deaths may have totaled between 50 million and 100 million.

From the 1950s onward the conditions for a new outbreak were becoming ever riper as increased movement across borders began. The movement was slowed by the cold war, during which travel in and out of communist countries was severely limited, but activity picked up again right afterward.

Like that period in the ancient past when cities emerged and the dense concentration of human population lead to devastating epidemics, now the number and distances of contacts among humans has reached a critical level. Severe Acute Respiratory Syndrome (SARS) demonstrated just how quickly a new disease can now move from one village in a corner of the world around the globe to dozens of other nations. The pneumonia-like illness originated in animals in rural China. During the outbreak in 2003, 8,100 people were infected and about 800 died. The disease started in a village in China and jumped to Hong Kong when a country doctor visited for a wedding. From the hotel he stayed in, the Metropole, about ten additional cases emerged and spread the disease to more than a dozen countries. The 2003 outbreak was halted when world alerts shut down travel in and out of China and Canada, two of the hot spots. Since that time more than a thousand new cases have been isolated in China, but few elsewhere. Just a few months of disease outbreak caused large economic losses. Because of the travel alarm the tourism industry lost an estimated $7.6 billion and 2.8 million jobs. The overall loss to China's economy in 2003 was $20.4 billion.

The time between when a microbe becomes able to successfully infect and kill human hosts to the time it *has* infected millions of people has dropped from decades to weeks. Such movement is virtually instantaneous in practical disease-fighting terms, because we have only a relatively small cadre of people around the world trying to spot and report the movement of new diseases.

We have watched in recent years as several horrifying new diseases have emerged. The Marburg virus was first identified in 1967 in Germany; since then there have been several outbreaks in Africa. The most recent one was still underway in Angola in May 2005, having killed more than three hundred people. About 90 percent of those infected have died.

Lassa fever started up in 1969 in Nigeria. Ebola appeared in 1976, and has taken several hundred victims in small outbreaks since. Legionnaire's disease emerged in 1976, and has since become a small, regular threat in certain urban spots. Lyme disease was discovered on the East Coast of the United States in 1977, but has since spread across the continent.

AIDS surfaced in New York and Los Angeles in 1981. It has since become the most generally threatening disease of humankind, as 40 million people are now infected with HIV, the virus that causes AIDS, and 5 million new infections appear every year. The total number killed since the beginning of the epidemic is about 20 million, and about 3 million deaths per year are now being recorded.

West Nile virus arrived in the United States in 1999, and within two years spread across the United States. It is a virus that is harbored by birds and spread to humans by mosquitoes. By the beginning of 2005 some 2,500 cases were reported in the United States, with 100 deaths and 900 cases of meningitis or encephalitis caused by West Nile. The virus is now permanently established in America.

Another recently identified mosquito-borne encephalitis is caused by the newly identified La Crosse virus. The disease was first recorded in the American Midwest in the 1960s, but in the 1990s began to spread. A few hundred cases are now reported annually, mostly in children.

Old familiar diseases are also making a comeback, often because our surveillance is so poor. Dengue fever is one of those diseases that hadn't been seen much in the United States for decades. The mosquito that carries it, *Aedes aegypti,* had been largely killed off by spraying and other programs in South, Central, and North America, but now it has gradually returned. The number of cases has gone up again: In the first few years of the 1980s, about eight hundred thousand cases were reported—more than double the number counted in the previous twenty-five years. In the second half of the 1980s the number continued upward, to over a million cases.

But the new dengue is different. It used to be a disease that produced a fever and a general weakness and malaise. But beginning in the 1950s a new type of dengue appeared, called dengue hemorrhagic fever. There are four different strains of the dengue virus that cause disease, and when one person is infected by more than one at a time, the lethal dengue hemorrhagic disease can result. It begins with a fever combined with joint and muscle pain; the fever continues for a week, but along the way it can suddenly cause bleeding from all the orifices and finally collapse of the circulatory system entirely. Over the past twenty years outbreaks of dengue hemorrhagic fever have increased both in number and severity as the mosquitoes have spread geographically.

By 1990, twenty-four cases had been recorded in the United States. The mosquito that carries dengue has now become a widespread inhabitant of the American South. But then, in 1985, a second mosquito carrier arrived in the Americas from Japan, in a shipment of used tires, as mentioned earlier. The mosquito which came with the tires was *Aedes albopictus*, the Asian tiger mosquito. (Used tires are a nearly ideal nursery for mosquitoes; they hold water in any position.) Both the Aegypti and the Asian tiger are now well established in the Southeastern United States, and they are able to carry not only dengue but viral encephalitis and yellow fever. In other words, the natural system to deliver these diseases is now in place.

For dengue, it was tires. For a cholera epidemic in 1991 it was bilge water. Cholera remains common in Asia, but had been largely eliminated from the Americas because water treatment had kept down the number of bacteria. But in the years before 1991 many towns in Peru cut down the amount of chlorine used to purify water. So when a ship from Asia arrived with bilge tanks full of cholera-contaminated water, and the ship emptied its ballast, the water of the port in Callao became contaminated. The fish and shellfish ingested the cholera, and then Peruvians picked it up in their diets and passed it through their plumbing into the water treatment plants. The germ survived, and returned to the taps in Callao as "clean" water. The first epidemic in almost a century was started, and it ran up through South America all the way to Mexico, causing four hundred thousand cases in one year.

In May 2005, the polio virus made a startling leap all the way from Nigeria to Indonesia, which hadn't had any cases in many years. As if to emphasize the political nature of disease, polio now occurs almost exclusively in Muslim areas in the world, because Muslims have resisted "Western" vaccination and the rich Muslim nations have failed to supply money or leadership for the antipolio campaign. Indonesia, the fourth largest nation in the world—and largest among Muslim nations—nevertheless had eliminated polio from within its border. But the rise of politically motivated resistance to immunization in Nigeria led to thousands of cases there. Initially twelve more African nations that had been free of the disease became reinfected. Then, on May 1, 2005, a case appeared again in Indonesia—a strain of the virus found in Nigeria. Now, the polio eradication campaign of the World Health Organization must track the small outbreaks in many more countries, even as it tries to finish off the two last regions that harbor hundreds of cases—Nigeria and northern India.

After September 11, the Bush administration provided more than $3 billion to build up American preparedness against the threat of terrorists using biological agents. Unfortunately, most of the money was shifted out of public health when it arrived in state coffers, or it was spent on preparing for the very unlikely occurrence of a biological attack by terrorists. Far less money was allocated to combating the much more likely scenario of a major naturally-occurring outbreak of one of the new or newly virulent diseases. Thus, the scientists of the academy reported in 2002 that the main threats from emerging diseases still had not been addressed.

The most feared disease among biologists and epidemiologists is not one of the forty or so new diseases identified in the past four decades. Strictly speaking, it is both new and old. It is the Avian flu, H5N1.

In 2005, the academy produced a warning—that of a pandemic of influenza may be imminent. If a virus like that of the 1918 epidemic were to appear today, the estimates of the number of deaths range from 2 million to 100 million worldwide. Remembering that SARS caused an international uproar and many billions of dollars in economic losses from only eight thousand infections and eight hundred deaths, it is easy to understand the worry of the biologists.

The 2005 report of the academy said, "Most infectious disease experts believe that the world stands on the verge of an influenza pandemic. Yet despite the legacy of the 1918 'Spanish flu' . . . the general public appears relatively unconcerned about the next 'killer flu.' Considerably more attention has been focused on protecting the public from terrorist attacks than from the far more likely and pervasive threat of pandemic influenza. . . . Meanwhile, the danger mounts as the world's capacity to produce vaccines shrinks and H5N1 reaches endemic levels in poultry in many parts of Asia."

Each of the previous killer flus started with strains that arose in birds: the 1918 epidemic that killed 40 million; the 1957 "Asian flu" epidemic that killed 1 million; and the 1968 "Hong Kong flu" epidemic that killed 4 million. The bird flu moving through Asia has already shown two of the three biological abilities needed to make a world pandemic: It has developed the ability to infect humans, and to kill them. It has not yet shown the ability to move from person to person, only from birds to people.

For Asia, the epidemic among chickens, ducks, and other birds is already a disaster, as tens of millions of birds have been killed by the flu and hundreds of millions more were destroyed as an emergency health measure to protect other birds and ultimately humans. In Thailand, the government compensates farmers for their losses in order to encourage poultry farmers to come forward when they have disease among their birds.

This points to one of the first problems of detecting an oncoming wave of deadly influenza—keeping track of viruses that are killing birds. The difficulty was highlighted by a recent case in California. In 2000, a flu strain called H6N2, which caused little illness in birds and was not counted as a human hazard, appeared in egg-laying chickens in southern California. There were about 15 million chickens raised in the region, and farmers realized that even though the virus was not thought to be hazardous to humans, just a mention that their birds were infected would be enough to create a huge drop in demand for their birds. So they kept quiet. Their commercial veterinarians followed the epidemic in the birds but did not report it to state officials. Only ten farms were involved at first, but as the secret was kept over the next two years, the virus spread to five more farms. A large outbreak occurred among birds in the town of Turlock, in northern California, where chickens from several states were taken to be slaughtered and processed. The virus spread from chickens to turkeys there. The spread became so intense, according to the academy report, that "the Turlock region, which is bound by three major highways, became known as the Triangle of Doom; a bird couldn't enter the area without becoming infected with H6N2." Eventually, the companies decided to clear up the epidemic and developed a plan to prevent further spread of the virus that does not penalize the farmers who allow their birds to be tested or immunized.

What is needed to prevent the worst damage from a human pandemic, the report said, is to: increase surveillance around the world;

replace disincentives for countries that report problems; create tests that detect early outbreaks; make possible the manufacture of vaccines and antiviral drugs to be used when an outbreak starts. So far, none of the above has been done.

The flu of 1918 killed 40 million in a year's time. That happened because the virus that causes the flu changes rapidly and once in a while becomes a rapid-spreading, more lethal variety. It happened in 1918, then again at large but somewhat less lethal scale in 1957 and 1968—when flu killed more than one hundred thousand in the United States alone. Because we have not continued vaccine research or pressed ahead with surveillance, if such an epidemic occurs now or in the next few years, the death toll might be as high as 100 million people.

The academy's 2002 report, which was entitled, "The Threat of Pandemic Influenza: Are We Ready?" was produced from several days of meetings among experts. Its bottom line came to this: "What can be said was echoed throughout the session—if the question is: 'Are we ready for a pandemic influenza?' the answer is 'no.'"

We know enough about the payoffs from preventive measures to know that the failure to do more can only be described as negligence. Most important, the cost of an outbreak is far larger than what it would have taken to prevent it. For example, it was estimated that in the decade from 1992 to 2002, the growth of GDP in thirty-three African countries declined by an average of 1.1 percent. By 2020, this will translate into a collective loss in just economic growth of 18 percent, or $144 billion. That's without counting medical costs, lost days at work, or the human cost of creating hundreds of thousands of orphans. Good surveillance work might well have averted a substantial portion of this damage.

Mad cow disease is a bomb waiting to go off in the United States and a number of other countries. Surveillance in the United States is weak because only a few cows are tested for it in a sampling procedure intended to catch the arrival of the disease. In one year, Britain lost more than $1.4 billion in beef sales when mad cow was identified there. The American industry is far larger, and the single near miss of a cow in Washington state a few years ago cost the beef industry $2 billion to $4 billion.

In 2002, two additional U.S. government reports were issued, and they described the urgency of the problem in a compelling new way: Deteriorating heath systems, combined with globalization, were now, they argued, a threat to U.S. national security. Any increase in human disease has large economic consequences, but there are also serious political consequences which follow as well.

One report was issued by the CIA as an unclassified version of their annual National Intelligence Estimate (NIE). The other was produced by national security specialists at the University of Maryland, the culmination of six years of work, and was titled, tellingly, the "State Failure Task Force Report." This linkage of health to national security was something new: Public health and foreign aid for health had never before been put so high on the security and foreign policy agendas.

These reports suggested that after the collapse of the Soviet Union, a world with a single superpower was in some ways *less* secure than a world of competing superpowers, and that public health was a vital element in the volatile mix. At the end of the cold war analysts inside and outside the American government had searched heaps of data for signs of trends that would determine the character of the new, emerging international order. Many political analysts in the late 1990s had looked forward to a world of greater peace and stability, with predictions of a new world order based on the principles of liberal democracy and the free market and managed by an international system.

Those predictions had failed to appreciate the rising role of the "nontraditional threats" highlighted by the CIA and University of Maryland studies. Those reports argued that the emergence of new diseases, the reemergence of old ones, and the decline in public health vigilance, combined with more and more contact between poor and wealthy nations, made it a near certainty that outbreaks in disease will increase. The rates of outbreaks and deaths from infectious diseases were already increasing in the United States after decades of decline, they pointed out, and the situations in some developing countries were much worse, especially in Africa, where HIV was decimating many countries' populations.

The NIE expressed the danger this way:

> *The dramatic increase in drug-resistant microbes, combined with the lag in the development of new antibiotics, the rise of megacities with severe health care deficiencies, environmental degradation, and the growing ease and frequency of cross-border movements of people and produce have greatly facilitated the spread of infectious diseases. . . . New and emerging infectious diseases will pose a rising global health threat, and will complicate U.S. and global*

security over the next 20 years. These diseases will endanger U.S. citizens at home and abroad . . . and exacerbate social and political instability in key countries and regions.

Both reports argued that the attempt to deal with the threat of disease outbreaks and subsequent economic and political trouble must begin immediately, because substantial time will be required to rebuild eroding international public health systems and to create new, global disease-prevention and -fighting institutions. "Development of an effective global surveillance and response system is at least a decade or more away," the report warned, "owing to inadequate coordination and funding at the international level, and lack of capacity, funds, and commitment in many developing and former communist states."

One thing about the state failure report and the NIE is especially convincing: They were both issued *before* September 11. Rereading them now, one can see with the benefit of hindsight that the threat of rising terrorism was in some way foreshadowed. After Osama bin Laden was expelled from Saudi Arabia, he moved to three different countries to carry on his terrorist activities—Afghanistan, Sudan, and Pakistan— all of which have qualified multiple times as failed states by the measures of the University of Maryland report. As the authors of that report emphasized, failed states are fertile breeding grounds for the discontent and rage that drives terrorism.

Terrorist leaders are not the desperate and abused poor; they are educated and have some means. Those whom they recruit are not quite so educated and well off, but they are not the dirt poor of the refugee camps either. The leaders and followers are not generally the ones suffering physically, but they depend upon the widespread impression of injustice and suffering around them. It is this impression of injustice, reinforced daily in the news, which drives their recruitment, and, more important, encourages the better off in their societies to turn a blind eye to the extreme tactics the militants use. The oxygen that fuels the fires of terrorism is the conviction in so many societies that injustice is being done.

This is why in addition to military action against terror, we must also address the issue of legitimacy directly. Doing so will require attending to the many pressing issues of public health in many nations.

The national security argument is, however, only one compelling justification for taking immediate and concerted action. Perhaps the most fundamental and unimpeachable argument of all is the moral one: It's the right thing to do.

Consider this fact: More than ten million children die each year from completely preventable causes. A mere handful of conditions are responsible for the vast majority of these deaths: pneumonia, diarrhea, measles, and malaria. Ironically, most of those who die could be saved with the cheapest and easiest of all treatments: routine vaccines, simple antibiotics, vitamin A, and insecticide-treated bed nets. These treatments cost a few cents to a dollar each.

In recent years, new methods of delivering aid have proved that it does not take batteries of outside experts or professionally trained workers to deliver the most basic interventions—they can be effectively delivered by volunteers, even in the most remote villages, even by the uneducated. Literally scores of innovative projects have been carried out in developing countries in recent years, and they are just the kind we need to back with far more aid dollars than we have given before.

Take one case in point. In Bangladesh, poor women were recruited to learn how to prepare and deliver an oral rehydration solution for children suffering from a catastrophic loss of fluid during diarrhea, one of the top killers of children on earth. The solution is made by a simple, though precise, recipe: a mixture of a bit of salt, a little sugar, and a cup of water. With just a little training the Bangladeshi mothers learned the techniques, and then volunteered to teach others. Over a period of a decade the skills became part of the local culture. The death rate from acute diarrhea was 50 percent before the effort; it dropped to less than 1 percent afterward. The project cost, in toto, about $9 million in aid. After its success, the women volunteers went on to work on other basics, such as the immunization and education of the poorest children. This project and subsequent ones inspired by it, which will be described later in the book, contributed to the remarkable rise in recent years of Bangladesh from a country with zero economic growth to over 5 percent growth annually. The country is still poor, it still has corruption, but it is now moving up.

Another successful intervention took place in seven countries of southern Africa. Picking up the lesson of South American nations, where measles had been eradicated, the countries of Botswana, Lesotho, Malawi, Namibia, South Africa, Swaziland, and Zimbabwe joined together in countrywide campaigns. They sent out teams of mobile volunteers, sometimes along with the local workers at village health posts, sometimes separately, working to vaccinate children between nine months and fourteen years old. Health clinics added measles to their regular vaccinations. Then the teams went back again to follow up. The projects succeeded in six of the seven countries, dropping the number of measles cases from 60,000 in 1996 to 117 in 2000, a near 100 percent success. The vaccinations cost $1.10 per child, and the majority of the cost was borne by the nations themselves, with some supplemental donor aid.

We can't afford to fail to make such effective investments in the health of the world's children. Apart from the practical value of health-and-wealth-creation, the children are innocent of the trouble in the world. They haven't had a chance to squander knowledge and good will and we should not waste it for them.

In the next chapters this book will describe several of these successful projects and how they demonstrate our ability to bring the fight for public health to a new, more effective level.

What is probably most remarkable about the current global health situation is a growing realization that we do in fact have the capability to end the worst of the world's health problems. A few decades ago that was impossible. The world is now considerably wealthier. In absolute numbers, there are fewer people in the worst poverty. The techniques and medicines needed are now available. Inexpensive ways of delivering them have been devised. What is needed now is the political will from the major donor nations, working with the poorest countries.

Which brings us from the arguments based on self-interest and altruism to those based on shared interest: A global effort at eradicating the worst health problems could trigger a significant economic boom in the receiving countries. Economist Jeffrey Sachs estimates that the savings from a global program would be $200 billion to $500 billion per year to start, and would add economic growth of several hundred billion more for the countries participating.

Until recent days, economists and politicians were skeptical that any such world program to deliver the most basic health interventions could work, or could be accommodated by the budgets of the major nations. But the issue isn't truly one of cost; it's one of building on discoveries made and hard-won knowledge attained, and of generating the political will to move ahead.

Fortunately, some leaders in health and economics have laid out clever, cost-effective plans for a new approach to global economic development, and several organizations have already been created to carry out those plans. The clear message put forward by the leaders of this developing movement is that the new approach must chiefly involve investment in human capital, with health as one priority.

The buzz is rising, the sound of a movement getting started. The stirring is in the United States, Europe, and elsewhere simultaneously. It seems to be a generational kind of movement, like a combination of the Marshall Plan and Peace Corps from previous generations, but on a bigger scale.

The names associated with one aspect or another of this movement cover an extraordinary range—from Bono to Bill Gates, George Bush to Jacques Chirac. It is early enough that the movement has no single name yet, only a growing number of people talking about it and what it might be able to do.

The plan of action being promoted might be referred to as a "new Marshall Plan" for wealthy countries to build up poorer countries, so that all can join in the coming globalization. Or it could be called a "global health movement," since the focus of its efforts to build up countries starts with carefully targeted interventions to stop the needless, easily preventable deaths and illnesses that still burden many countries around the world.

Groups putting energy into the discussion, and sounding nearly like they are on the same page, range from the Central Intelligence Agency and the Rand Corporation to Oxfam and the Global Vaccine Initiative. Those stepping forward include both multinational corporations and small antipoverty groups. The ideas loosely bound together by this movement are inspiring, fairly bold, and distant enough from divisive politics to get even longtime foreign aid critic Senator Jesse Helms saying he has been inspired by something Bono said. Talk about the movement has been further stirred up by rock concerts like Live Aid (and as this is being written, "Live 8") and those generating tsunami relief from around the world.

This coalescing movement reaches down into economics and history for its rationale and takes advantage both of globalization and recent work done in economics, and of breakthroughs from recent successful health and development projects in Asia and Africa. The ideas are well-founded and deeply compelling, and the need is urgent.

But is such a global program really plausible? Haven't we been throwing money at underdeveloped countries for years and getting terribly disappointing results?

The public may as yet be skeptical about the value and practicality of this global initiative. But we must remember just how extraordinary our achievements in the past have been when we have devoted concerted effort and adequate funds to the goal.

Probably the best way to appreciate the scale of the achievements realized when we applied ingenuity and adequate public funds is to start by taking the longer view of history. Consider the extraordinary rise in human prospects in the past 150 years. We have built health and wealth unlike anything in history; the question now is whether to continue the progress or fall back to preglobal times.

For all of human history the shadow at our backs has been the specter of illness and death, and it has for us the most terrifying features. It may come at any time, at any age. We cannot see the shadow approach, but instead it reaches out from behind a curtain, unexpected. It has the power to give us just a passing fever, or instead to pull us entirely out of our place in the world, to erase us from all concern. From before historical time, we have tried to conjure this specter away.

We alone among the animals, it seems, know we are going to die. It was as if, in exchange for our sentience, we must live with the specter of death. We can see the worry present even in prehistoric sites. There are burial places tens of thousands of years old, where seeds and stones are set in a pattern—the remnants of ornaments we arrayed with our dead. Calendars were laid in graves. This poor debris already suggested signs of resistance to our fate. The muffled voices rise from the ground: We are not just flesh, and we refuse to go away! We have invoked the gods; we have given extra deference to the shamans who tried to save us. Beyond the prayer and sacrifice, we have always tried practical measures as well. The earliest evidence of medicine comes from Shanidar in prehistoric Persia, where traces of medicinal drugs used forty thousand years ago have been unearthed.

About six thousand years ago we began to write of our worry about sickness and death. Writers in Mesopotamia and Egypt describe not a few but hundreds of medical procedures and drugs that had been employed long before their use was recorded. In one Egyptian papyrus, 876 remedies made of 500 different substances were delineated—and this was three thousand years before the "ancient" Greek culture gave us Hippocrates.

But the results of one hundred thousand years of incantation and medicine came to little. For all of those seven thousand generations in which humans went from hunting to settling and then to full culture, the fundamental fact of life was not altered: At birth, humans could expect, on average, to live to be about twenty-five to thirty-five years old. In "civilized" England in 1800 the average length of life had not changed since the time of ancient Egypt.

Then, with the coming of the last globalization, something *did* change, and the change was both quick and dramatic. So profound were the gains in public health made within the span of about a century that this period, from approximately the middle of the nineteenth century to the middle of the twentieth, is often referred to as the "vital revolution." For many, this health revolution brought forth a literal defeat of death. Average life expectancy around the world rose from about twenty-five to thirty years in 1800 to forty-seven years in 1950, rose again to sixty-seven years by 2004. The gains were not confined to the West. In China, life expectancy rose from forty to sixty-three years during the same period. It rose similarly in India, and even more in Japan. In the most developed countries it reached sixty-six years in 1950 and eighty years in 2004.

In graphic terms, at about A.D. 1800 the average age at death remained unchanged from ten thousand years before. The increase in human population shows a similar pattern, with the number of people on the planet rising only very slowly from about 6000 B.C. to A.D. 1800. Then, both figures started suddenly shooting up, in an almost vertical line, roughly between 1800 and 1900. After thousands of generations, suddenly, in about five generations, human life was transformed. It is as if the chart stopped tracking one species and shifted to another.

Robert Fogel, a Nobel Prize–winning economist who has spent a lifetime trying to understand this sudden break, has written that the change was in fact a rapid evolution. But it was not genetic; it was cultural. We were, across the globe, a different people in A.D. 2000 than we had been only a handful of generations before. Our lifetimes suddenly doubled and trebled, and not just in the wealthy countries. Demographer James Riley says that in 1800 there were about one billion people on the planet who would live to less than thirty years old; by 2000, there were six billion who would live to be almost seventy years old, and the ramp of the line is still slanting upward.

During recent generations, Fogel wrote, "human beings have gained an unprecedented degree of control over their environment—a degree of control so great that it sets them apart not only from all other species, but from all previous generations of *Homo sapiens*." The gain was not only in health and longevity, but vitality; human body size is now 50 percent greater, and the number of hours a person can work beyond bare survival and lethargy has increased many hours per day. Taking England as an example, Fogel wrote that the increase in nutrition and energy, combined with our newly efficient ways of turning that into work, accounts for about half of all the economic growth of England from 1790 to the present.

Health is the crowning achievement of modern humankind, said James Riley, surpassing wealth, military power, or political stability in import. Of the three great social edifices built by humans—the infrastructures of government, economy, and health—the institutions of health have been the most successful,

> *delivering a larger quantity of long life to a larger share of the world population than politics have delivered good government or economies wealth. . . . Never before has such a large share of the human population been able to live long enough for people to frame a mature sense of themselves, to see their children grow up, even to get to know their grandchildren. Never before have so many people been able confidently to anticipate their own survival into old age. This achievement is a spectacular demonstration of the human capacity to manage itself.*

Though people tend to think of the pharmaceutical revolution as most important in reducing mortality, 80 percent or more of the life expectancy gains actually came from sanitation such as clean drinking water and separate sewage, and from the understanding of disease transmission which led to hand washing and medical antisepsis.

New drugs have contributed only a relatively small part. For example, 80 percent of tuberculosis was eliminated between 1845 and 1945; that was *before* penicillin. But the new medicines did combine potently with the vital revolution already underway, and the two began to work in tandem.

The vital revolution began with the dogged efforts of a cadre of reformers called the "sanitarians." In England, they included Thomas Southwood Smith, John Simon, William Farr; in France, they were led by Louis Rene Villerme and Pierre Louis; in Germany, by Rudolf Virchow and Johann Frank; in the United States by William Welch, Hermann Biggs, William Park, and others. They strove to force towns to deliver decent living conditions for workers. A chief item on the agenda was to deliver clean water to neighborhoods and take sewage away separately. They wanted streets cleaned and rooming houses opened to ventilation. The sick shed the particles of disease, so the healthy must keep an antiseptic distance: Washing with soap after contact is vital, and washing before preparing food no less so. We must take care not to use water that contains the effluents of others. The principles are simple, but in crowded societies they are not easy to put in place, either in the home or in the city water and sewage systems. It took more than a hundred years to sell the educated inhabitants of the globe on the need to invest in the necessary infrastructure for following these mandates on the large scale.

At the same time a complementary movement got underway to use the body's own defenses—through vaccines—to combat a number of the most elemental diseases. This effort reached a memorable moment in 1955, when the largest human experiment in history was completed to test the polio vaccine. The vaccine succeed in protecting against polio, and on the day the experimental proof was announced it was greeted in the United States with bells ringing from church steeples and town councils declaring laudatory and self-congratulatory resolutions. The people in most countries of the world had accepted the notion that health had become a cooperative public venture, a matter for society and common interests; they not only accepted the notion, but avidly supported the efforts. The crowning achievement of this global public health movement was the eradication of smallpox, which required fourteen years of labor in two hundred countries. The last natural case of the disease was recorded in 1977.

Scholars now call the period between 1944 and 1973 the "golden age" of prosperity and public health. One of the great ironies of the "crowning achievements" racked up during those years, however, was that they led to a false sense of security, and to complacency. After the vanquishing of polio in America, one scientist had predicted with satisfaction, "There are diseases that offer threats, but, over all, in the field of infectious ones, most of the killing ones are under control. . . . Man one day may be armed with vaccine shields against every infectious ill that besets him." In September 1978, after smallpox had been eliminated, health ministers and leaders of the world's nations met in Alma-Ata, Kazakhstan. The language of their declaration was confident, almost euphoric. The delegates reflected on the rise of health and prosperity and declared that it could and should be extended to all, down to the poorest of the poor. They said that health was a fundamental "human right" and that the gap between the rich and poor countries was "politically, morally and economically unacceptable." Health "for all" could be achieved, in great part, by the millennium in 2000, they said.

How, then, after such a remarkable set of achievements, do we find ourselves at such a crucial pivot point today, where the disease threat has gained so much traction against our defenses? Why did the backslide happen?

It happened because the golden age of achievement was followed by the era of forgetting. The grand public enterprises that had defeated disease gradually fell out of favor.

First, the success of a century of public health campaigns, followed by the creation of miracle drugs such as antibiotics, led to overconfidence. Scientists and doctors had defeated infectious disease, and the victory was expected to be permanent. Lulled into a sense of complacency in the industrial world, and most especially in the United States, governments and citizens began to spend more and more money on personal health care and less on public health protections such as disease surveillance and vaccine research.

"We spend vast sums to lengthen the lives of terminally ill patients by a few days," wrote physician and essayist Ronald Glasser, speaking of the pattern of recent decades. "And we refuse to make modest investments that would prevent millions of needless illnesses and deaths."

"The great public-health victories of the nineteenth century and early twentieth centuries over yellow fever, cholera, encephalitis, smallpox, puerperal fever, and a host of other infectious diseases," Glasser wrote, "were largely the result of preventive measures enacted by visionary public officials: improved sanitation and nutrition (safe water and food, decent housing, paved streets, sewers), vigorous powers of quarantine to prevent contagion, mosquito control and the installation of window glass, and the creation of vaccination programs."

But

for the last quarter century, especially after the election of Ronald Reagan and his declaration that government itself is the problem that afflicts us, the public-health infrastructure of this country has been eviscerated. Between 1981 and 1993, public-health expenditures declined by 25 percent as a proportion of overall health spending; in 1992, less than 1 percent of all American health-care spending was devoted to public health. That trend has continued, even after the anthrax attacks of 2001, when politicians suddenly realized how vulnerable the nation was to biological attack. Overall, thirty-two states cut their public-health budgets between fiscal years 2002 and 2003. . . . In fact, the President's 2005 budget . . . cuts $1.1 billion from the "Function 550" account which finances disease-prevention programs and other public-health initiatives.

In this era citizens and even scientists appeared to forget our fundamental biology, which tells us that organisms will adapt to new environs and evolve new abilities to continue multiplying their numbers. We cannot actually expect to defeat biological organisms; once defeated they will always change and reemerge. Organisms living in isolated populations of animals in jungles will readily break out when their territory is penetrated by people.

When AIDS appeared, an entirely new disease on the scale of his-torical killers, the first reaction from the leaders in America and Eu-rope was tragically not one of drawing together for the common good, but of silence. Worse, there was sotto voce muttering that those who got the disease did so because of their own sins. In the United States it was seven years before the president even acknowledged the existence of the epidemic. As the epidemic ramped up, the budget for the Food and Drug Administration (FDA) was actually cut, not increased. Dur-ing the 1980s, the federal government in America took large health programs, cut their funding, and then turned them over to the states to operate. Funds for world programs—and for the United Nations itself—became contentious; health budgets slipped downward in pri-ority. The largest county health systems in America, by the 1990s, faced outright bankruptcy.

The decline in public spending in the United States and to a degree in Europe was broad. The figures that characterize a nation's health best, however, are not budgets. They are mortality statistics. Because they do not fluctuate much year to year they are the most reliable guides to where we were headed. By the 1980s those trends began to fall for the first time in memory. For example, the number of people in the United States who die from infectious diseases—a sign of century-long progress—went down through 1980. In that year it reached an all-time low. Then it turned and headed back up, increasing 5 percent per year until now. By the end of the 1990s the number had doubled to 170,000 per year.

The splendid world progress in life expectancy also began to stall in the 1980s; it dropped in fifty-one countries of Africa and Asia for the first time in decades. In Botswana, for example, life expectancy was as high as sixty-three, and would have gone up to seventy-two if it were not for AIDS. It has dropped to thirty-nine years and is expected to fall to twenty-seven in the next decade. In the United States the decline in the rate of infant mortality, possibly the best final indicator of progress—or lack of it—also stalled. In 2002, it even dropped, the first time that had happened since 1958. In the 1950s the United States had been among the top nations in that measure—sixth in the world. But by 2002 the U.S. ranking had slipped to forty-first among nations. Some demographers have predicted a drop in American life expectancy as well—and soon. If that occurs it would be for the first time since the nineteenth century.

In the past several years economists, foreign policy experts, and leaders in public health have produced a growing body of articles and books seeking to understand the challenges we are facing and how we can meet them. They have begun to sketch ways forward, which will be introduced in more detail in later chapters. The plans put forth are ambitious, but the vital lesson to be learned from the stories of the new generation of low-cost, innovative health projects is that those plans are practical and entirely achievable. The essential extra ingredient is that public support for these plans must be mobilized.

At the United Nations Millennium Summit in 2000 the member nations agreed to a set of specific goals and timetables to combat poverty, disease, illiteracy, and environmental degradation. Most of the emphasis was on bolstering health in poor countries, reducing deaths of children under five by two-thirds, reducing maternal death by three-quarters, and reversing the spread of major diseases, especially AIDS, tuberculosis, and malaria. After the goals were outlined a consulting commission, called the Millennium Development Project—led by economist Jeffrey Sachs of Columbia University—set out to devise plans whereby the goals could be reached. Within this framework for raising money for specified goals, there are a number of powerful new ideas about how to get the money to the poor countries. The main financial mechanism is the newly created Global Fund to Fight AIDS, Tuberculosis and Malaria. It is independent of the United Nations and operates in an entrepreneurial mode—that is, it gives grants but demands accountability and progress toward specific health targets, such as increasing the number of people who get basic treatments or achieving lower death rates. President Bush has set up two parallel projects, the Millennium Challenge Account, which operates in a fashion similar to the Global Fund, and the $15 billion President's Emergency Plan for AIDS Relief.

There is general agreement among experts who have studied the challenges of the current world situation that spending on aid, particularly health, must be massively increased, and that the way to spend the money is by providing grants to strictly results-oriented projects.

In July 2005, the G8 group of nations promised to double their aid to poor nations; the promise was an encouraging step forward, though the amounts pledged were not by themselves enough to have a major effect on disease and poverty.

Clearly, as we find ourselves facing the many dangers posed by the jet-fueled processes of globalization, we must generate the public will to confront those challenges, beginning with support for the new global health movement. The slippage of recent years need not be permanent. In fact, we have never been in a better position to consolidate our previous gains and move on to add health and wealth around the world. Remarkably, in each field needed to build a surge of health and consequent development, we have made great strides forward—from the economics of development based on health, to the details of how to deliver results on the ground in some of the most difficult places on earth. The time to act is now; the consequences of not acting will be grave.

The stories of these various projects and the driven individuals who have devoted their lives, often times over many years, to getting them off the ground are profoundly inspiring.

There is the story of the Bangladeshi born ex–Shell Oil executive who committed himself to helping rebuild his devastated country, and invented a new breed of home-grown aid agency now often referred to as "the world's greatest NGO," which, by sponsoring ingeniously designed, inexpensive projects has helped to raise life expectancy in the country from forty-four to sixty-three years. There is the story of a grand experiment in AIDS prevention undertaken in Botswana, one of the nations most profoundly affected by the disease, that has produced such success that twelve other African countries have now followed its lead. In India, there is the story of a dogged campaign to search out and vaccinate every last child against polio, being executed one door knock at a time by an army of volunteers. And in Nepal, with some of the worst rates of poverty and child mortality in the world, there is the astonishing story of the grandmothers who, empowered with the responsibility to administer simple doses of vitamin A to children in their villages, have helped avert an estimated two hundred fifty thousand child deaths a year in the country. This program has been hailed as among the simplest and most cost-effective ways to save lives ever devised.

The stories of these programs will be told in the next chapters, to bring to life the remarkable potential of the kind of more measured, low-tech, home-administered, largely volunteer-run, and carefully monitored projects that aid must be provided for. Many other projects might have been selected—there is a host of good examples—but these are the stories that spoke to me most powerfully as I traveled around the world researching this book. They speak volumes about the enormous strides we can make if we will only devote the necessary attention and resources to the task at this critical moment. I do not believe one can read these stories and come away without the deep conviction that the time is right, and the tools are in place, for a new vital revolution.

PART ONE

Splendidly Simple Solutions

1

A Pinch, A Fist, A Cup of Water

Bangladesh Rises

At its base, any proposal to greatly increase aid to poor countries will depend upon a belief that the projects will have good results. Unfortunately, for many years, foreign aid efforts have been subjected to caustic criticism, and too many projects have deserved it. But it is wrong to say that we have learned nothing in the past fifty years of administering aid to the developing world, or that we cannot run successful projects now if we have good leaders for the work. That is no longer a responsible argument. There are simply too many first-rate aid projects on the record over the past two decades for those objections to hold up. Models have emerged to guide the way about how money can be best directed, and perhaps no such model is more impressive than that developed by the Bangladeshi businessman who returned home to help save his country.

Fazle Hasan Abed, when he was growing up in Bangladesh, dreamed of building ships. After training for that, he eventually realized that not too many ships were going to be built in Bangladesh, and

settled on the more likely career of accountancy. After a British education he joined Shell Oil, and rose rapidly to become a top accounting
executive by his early thirties.

Then, politics and history pulled his career out from under him.
On the night of November 12, 1970, the Indian Ocean conspired to
end his career as an international executive.

There was a full moon over the Bay of Bengal on that night. That
meant the tide was already high when a storm roared up the bay, driving it even higher. It was a cyclone, massively broad and throwing
winds more than 150 miles per hour and tidal surges up to twenty feet
high. But it was not the breadth of the storm or its wind speed that
eventually put it above all other storms; it was what followed. U.S.
forecasters saw it coming, and government forecasters in what was
then East Pakistan saw it. Notice never reached the people where it
would strike the next day, November 13. The counting is still vague,
though it is believed that five hundred thousand people, maybe more,
died in that storm—the worst in recorded human history.

Bangladesh was already in turmoil—both political and social—
when the great storm arrived. Leaders were pushing for independence
from Pakistan. When the storm arrived President Yahya Khan, who
lived a thousand miles away in wealthier western Pakistan, ignored it.
Instead, he flew on a junket to China. It was a turning point in history;
the revolt against him soon began, and within months all-out war between East and West in Pakistan had started. After a startling rampage
of rape and slaughter by the western troops, India intervened and
helped push the West Pakistani troops out.

Out of this double catastrophe Bangladesh was born, an independent and utterly devastated state. And with the independence also was born a small group of well-educated Bangladeshis who went to the villages and borders to give aid to the victims of the storm and the war. Ten million refugees who had fled to India and Burma were now streaming home to villages that no longer existed.

For Fazle Abed, it was the end of one life, the start of another. He had been living both in Europe and in Bangladesh comfortably; now he could see his country ruined, yet struggling to be born. He happened to be in Europe and quickly went home to help. "Two years," he thought, "or maybe a few more." Abed once described the moment to a reporter: "I was suddenly confronted with the massive death and destruction after the cyclone. It was a life-changing experience, immediately followed by the political turmoil." Then, as he began the work of building Bangladesh back up, he said, "It was a continuous process of questioning your own existence, and the kind of life you lead."

That was a third of a century ago now. Fazle Abed never went back to his job in international business. He began with refugee work, carting bamboo for houses, supplying tools for workers, and organizing medical aid. But as he worked, month by month, and then year by year, he was drawn farther in. He could see that Bangladesh, while it was dirt poor, was nevertheless united by language and culture and religion; a completely new start was just possible, building on the glories of ancient Bengali culture, known for it high-mindedness, its poetry, its music and art.

Mr. Abed often wears dark suits, his face is mahogany brown, and above it all floats a shock of all-white hair. He wears rimless spectacles. His face is round, gentle, and almost cherubic. Journalists coming through have said his gentle demeanor makes him seem like a holy man without the robes, or maybe a Mother Teresa who can count and manage.

His office is in a building that is among the tallest in the country—it's nineteen floors—and he points through the window to the sprawling city of Dhaka below. There are 13 million people in the city, pressed cheek by jowl in one of the greatest encampments of the poor in the world. Next to his office is a narrow lake. On one shore are modern roads, apartments, and shops, and from his window you can see the corrugated tin shacks jammed in rows along the other shore, so close to one another it is hard to walk between them. "Look there," he says, "We have *shastyo shebiko* [health workers] in that neighborhood. We started with the rural areas, but now we are in the city. Two for every one in the rural areas are needed in the city."

Accountant Abed is now nearing seventy years old and he is the head of an organization that has become well known among those who work in the teeming field now called "development." It is the field you go into when you want to build society from the bottom. Among organizations that do this work, the one led by Mr. Abed is actually more than just famous; it is in danger of becoming a legend. It has even been referred to as "the world's greatest NGO."

Here is the accountant's-eye view, just the basic numbers, on its work since those days after the storm and the war of independence.

It is the largest nongovernmental organization in any developing country. It started with six people (Abed and five friends) who borrowed $300,000 dollars from family and others who sympathized with refugee care. The group had no intention of staying with the

46

work, or of growing larger. But as the government of the new na-tion was unable to muster all the effort needed, the duties and op-portunities kept coming to the little group that gave itself the name (remember, he's an accountant) Bangladesh Rural Advancement Committee.

Now, from six people, the BRAC has 146,000 workers. Over the years, it is said, BRAC has become so large and powerful that it is in fact a parallel government within Bangladesh, though it has actively avoided trying to become that. It has taken on three basic missions for the rural poor: first, a few key health services; second, primary schooling for dropouts; and third, microfinancial services for poor vil-lagers. It has intentionally limited its work to the poor only. (BRAC discovered that providing services for all made it certain that the bet-ter off would swamp demand and push out the poor.) Its work was limited largely to women, who also ran the programs in villages. (BRAC learned that offering services to women gave their efforts great leverage—women and children were the worst served but the most likely to benefit from health, schooling, and small loans.)

Still, BRAC is a large and potent organization, touching in some way the lives of about half the country's people every day. The origi-nal intent was to try to help build the nation from the bottom up. Now, after three decades, it is difficult to say what proportion of progress in Bangladesh is due only to BRAC. Many other groups have been begun as well, and the government shoulders a substantial part of the burden, as do charities and commercial companies.

However the parts are added up, Bangladesh has far outstripped all predictions for its future. In the 1970s, when referring to the dregs, the worst in the world, it was usual to mention Bangladesh. American secretary of state Henry Kissinger publicly called it, "a basket case."

About that time, deaths of children under five stood at 248 dead for every 1,000. Because each woman was having, on average, about seven children, this meant every mother probably lost at least one. But by 2003 the death rate among young children had dropped by more than two-thirds, from 248 to 69 per 1,000. As the children were saved, and as family planning methods were made available, families then decided to limit their growth. Family size went from about seven children per family in 1970 to three per family now.

In 1970, a baby born in Bangladesh could expect, on average, to live about forty-four years. Today babies can expect sixty-three years of life. And that life will be in a different environment. Bangladesh was one of the few countries in history where women had lower life expectancies than men; that has reversed. In 1970, boys went to school and girls stayed home—now both are educated in the same numbers. Literacy has doubled, from 26 percent to more than 51 percent. Polio was eradicated in Bangladesh years before it was eliminated from India, Pakistan, and many other, wealthier countries. The rate of economic growth at the end of the 1960s and in the early 1970s fluttered not far above zero. It has now run above 5 percent per year for a decade. The country was importing food; now it can more than feed itself, and three-quarters of the economy has turned to other business.

Among the most interesting figures about BRAC is the one for donations. BRAC started with gifts totaling about $300,000 from local families. International donors later began to chip in. By 1994, BRAC had a budget of about $64 million; 72 percent of it came from international donors. But the idea was not to take handouts forever. BRAC weaned itself away, and by 2004 BRAC had a budget of $235 million, and only 20 percent of it came from donors. The rest was raised by BRAC programs themselves with its own workers' enterprises and sales. It might be tempting to think that an antipoverty program might even turn a profit, but BRAC is satisfied to produce 80 percent of its needed resources.

The first BRAC programs—and the most famous—are the health programs. That is probably because their outcomes are measured in lives rather than dollars or years in school. It is also because the BRAC village workers carried out the single greatest "technology transfer" in history, though it is little noted in the West. Researchers, first in other parts of the world, then crucially in laboratories in Dhaka and Calcutta, had discovered the key to the deadly diarrheas that come with the age-old plagues of cholera, rotavirus, shigella, and *E. coli*. With an accountant's care and a revolutionary zeal, the BRAC workers proved that a medicine used for decades in intravenous solution in hospitals to save babies could be made at home—and used there successfully by women who were illiterate. Against the advice of doctors, and under the cloud of regular attacks, their scientifically rigorous tests proved the method. Then they began a ten-year-long project to teach the mothers of Bangladesh how to make and use the lifesaving solution. Using it, the death rate for babies with severe diarrhea dropped from 50 percent to less than 1 percent.

House by house, in its first years the volunteers trained thirteen million women in the techniques, beginning in 1979. Now, after more than two decades of working the villages the method has simply been absorbed as part of Bengali culture. The method, called oral rehydration therapy (ORT), eventually caught on elsewhere and is now being spread worldwide under the official aegis of the World Health Organization. It is credited with saving more than a million babies every year around the world. And world figures reflect the change: In 1970, more than five million babies died each year of diarrheal disease worldwide; by 2003, two million were dying of it.

BRAC health workers, at the request of the government, also worked on delivering basic immunization. There are cheap vaccines for six diseases that children get, and in Bangladesh in the 1980s only about 2 percent of the population got them. After the BRAC and government work, the figure rose rapidly to over 65 percent, and now about 80 percent of Bangladeshi children get immunized.

Progress against disease and poverty comes not only from smart work and organization on the ground. It also comes from science and technology. Poverty workers sometimes complain that basic science gets too much glory and money, while the people on the ground are actually making the progress one spadeful at a time.

But both are necessary, and in Bangladesh, like everything else jammed together, they work side by side in the same buildings, the same rooms, and sometimes in the same person. As one former diarrhea researcher there put it, the job was to "take the science to where the diarrhea is."

At the time of the first worldwide cholera epidemics, scientists, statisticians, and politicians were just beginning to use figures and graphs to see the big picture in human health and wealth. It soon was clear that in times of great trouble human anguish becomes centered in the bowels. During disasters like hurricanes and wars and in the most neglected places on the planet the condition that seizes the moment is diarrhea.

To Western ears it sounds like something from the past. Deadly diarrhea is caused by a variety of organisms, and to us they have an antique sound—cholera, rotavirus, shigella. But they are deeply embedded in our language. The guts are the seat of courage and of our fundamental moods; melancholia, the evocative term for depression, comes from the "black bile" of the gut that was thought to cause it. In the Bible the psalmist says his bowels instruct him what to do, saying his inward conviction issues from them, and when Joseph ran to his brother, the text says that he made haste because his bowels did "yearn upon his brother." Elizabeth I in asserting her authority said, "I know I have the body of a weak, feeble woman, but I have the heart and stomach of a king, a king of England, too." When Shakespeare was speaking of political trouble he called up images of the innards: "Civil dissension is a viperous worm that gnaws the bowels of the commonwealth."

All this because the gut is one of the more vulnerable parts of the anatomy. The digestive tract is a remarkable organ system, in the shape of a skin hose that can deftly separate water, chemicals, and nutrients, absorbing the required while flushing out the unneeded.

That is where the heroism in development begins. Researchers for years puzzled through the strange central event of diarrhea—that the intestine which usually absorbs water and nutrients suddenly changes in disease, at the level of individual bowel cells, and reverses their flow. They not only reject new fluids coming by, but dump out their own inside fluids, ultimately causing a total collapse of tissue walls and bloodstreams. The body is mostly water; during these events a massive internal drought breaks down the structures in the body and forces the heart and other organs to stop. Research eventually focused on the receptor molecules that dot the outsides of cells, and on how they were controlling the entry and exit of salts called electrolytes.

Some of the key work was done in Calcultta and in the Cholera Research Laboratory in Dhaka. (It is still there, and is now called the International Centre for Diarrhoeal Disease Research, Bangladesh. In fact, after the slashing of international public health funds in the 1980s and 1990s, it is the *only* major international research lab left standing in the developing world, after years when labs dotted the continents. Now, with a large HIV laboratory in Botswana, it is hoped a new cycle of research in developing countries is starting up.)

In principle, by the 1970s, the physiology was clear. Cells of the intestine must keep a balance of water and salt inside and outside themselves to carry on working. Some disease organisms, in an effort to get themselves spread from one person to another, have evolved the ability to create a huge flushing action of water by attacking receptors on the outside of intestinal cells, breaking down the inside-outside balance and turning the cells into outward-only pumps. Until these crucial years of research, it was thought that during disease cells could only dump their water, not absorb more at the same time. But the research proved there were two pumps available on the cells, and if the cells were given fluids with sugar in them, the second set of pumps would start working to take in water while the other pumps were still flushing it out. This was the key—sugar to get cells to stop the one-way outflow, and salt to get the normal operational levels back.

In hospitals it is possible to pump enough fluid into a cholera patient using an intravenous tube. But trying to translate this hospital procedure to the field was difficult.

In fact, the first real experiment with the idea was disastrous. Robert Phillips, working during a cholera epidemic in the Philippines, tried giving a simple sugar-saltwater solution to patients by mouth. All were very sick, but five of thirty quickly died. His solution had too much salt, and the experiment killed the patients before the disease got them. Phillips was mortified. He began to think such field-rough treatment for diarrhea would never be possible. A few years later, he found himself the director of the Cholera Research Laboratory in Dhaka just as new discoveries on the physiology of diarrhea were made, ones that hinted at what might have saved his earlier patients. But he could not bring himself to approve further life-threatening experiments. As it happened, though, a small satellite clinic of the Cholera Research Laboratory came under different funding and jurisdiction than Phillips's main laboratory. It was in Matlab village, south of Dhaka. Scientists there wanted to go ahead; Phillips agreed to not try to stop them if they worked in Matlab.

The doctors there felt they had to try again. After all, during the years of crises in Bangladesh the tragedy was painfully clear—children in the villages were dying in waves. A lucky few near hospitals got intensive Western-style intravenous drips. It involved getting a doctor's diagnosis as to severity, and a nurse to get a bag of expensive intravenous fluid into the patient's arm with a sterile syringe, then someone to monitor the flows and progress.

At bottom, though, it seemed that the difference between the living and the dead was just some sugar and saltwater. The multiplication of cholera bacteria or rotavirus in the gut would gradually stop on its own. But the loss of fluid caused in the first day of illness was what killed the children. Replacing fluids was the key.

The turning point came with a couple of experiments. In one at the Cholera Research Laboratory, patients were started on intravenous drips, and then switched to oral fluids. The experiment showed they could eliminate the need for 80 percent of the IV fluid and setups. Then, during 1971, in one refugee camp in West Bengal when a cholera epidemic was cutting down children, a doctor from Calcutta took the next step, out of necessity. As the patients around him were facing death, he couldn't even start with IVs. He gave homemade solutions to patients entirely by mouth, a sip at a time and with the right salts, until the worst danger had passed. It worked.

So in Bangladesh and India, the answer was in the air. The labs where the scientific work was being done were in the same building where the children were dying by the hundreds, and that alone moved the work to the next possibility. Fazle Abed and his assistance workers knew the scientists as well, and had followed the work.

It was then, in 1979, that the BRAC group met to talk about increasing the size of its health work from a few villages to the greater part of the entire nation. They did not want to try to deliver too much;

they decided to pick one intervention, one treatment that would make the most difference.

This was the 1970s; modern Western technology and medicine were greatly desired, while local products and technologies were denigrated. Medical authorities in Dhaka, the capital of Bangladesh, as well as authorities from the World Health Organization, were actively opposed to treating deadly diarrhea with homemade solutions in the hands of local women. Though it had been proven in lab work and shown in emergencies, it was not credible that village people could take over and use this medical technology. In fact, they said, it would be irresponsible to depend on illiterate women for such medical care. And they were right in a way; there was a serious problem. A study in the United States had shown that fully trained nurses, when taught how to make the oral rehydration solution in a lecture class, often failed to get it right. If they couldn't do it, how could village women?

If mothers were to treat severe diarrhea, they had to know when to act, how to make the lifesaving liquid, and how to administer it. The liquid, in medical terms, was a "balanced electrolyte solution for rehydration." It was mostly water, with some sugar and a small amount of salt. But the proportions had to be correct. If it was too salty, it would accelerate the fluid loss and kill the infants instead of saving them. If it contained too little sugar, it would be ineffective, as if no treatment at all was given. Some researchers at the Cholera Research Laboratory in Dhaka, and at the Indian Council for Medical Research in Calcutta, now believed they knew more about how to get it right—just the right mixture and just the right delivery.

While the argument among medical people was going on, the BRAC group was ready to build a health campaign in the villages.

Abed led the discussion at BRAC over what to attack, and how—the diseases killing the most were pneumonia, diarrhea, measles, tuberculosis, and tetanus. Which one could be attacked most successfully? Diarrhea looked like their best chance because of the possibility that they might be able, as John Rohde of ICD said at the time, to "take the science to where the diarrhea is."

For the BRAC leaders, as they sat in the village of Sulla in rural Bangladesh discussing their strategy, it was clear that the high death rate from diarrhea would continue. They walked through the problems.

Bags of saline were sold by local doctors in Bangladesh, but the price was one hundred taka per bag, and five to ten bags would be needed to treat each patient. At the time, the average income in the villages was about fifteen hundred taka per family per year, and the average child had three bouts of serious diarrhea per year, so the bags could quickly bankrupt a family. Packets of soluble salts were also beginning to be manufactured—couldn't they be mixed at home? They were cheaper than saline, and in theory could be sold in Bangladeshi villages, where the women would then buy them in emergencies, take them home, and mix them in water to give to their sick babies. But no distribution system was in place, and if the government were to buy the packets for distribution, it would take hundreds of millions of packets to cover the country. And in the end, would the marketed packets reach the ones who needed them most? The instructions on the packets might or might not be clear; but in any case, 80 percent of the women intended to use them were illiterate. And finally, even with relatively inexpensive packets, it would still have to be the mothers who would diagnose the problem, buy the salts, mix them in water at home, and give the solution to their babies.

It was clear that the center of the problem were questions about the mothers, not the solution. Why not acknowledge it and deal with it?

"From the beginning we had this sense that you must trust people," said Abed. "Trust the mothers. We had a great belief that illiterate people, any human beings, trained to do certain things could be very good at it. Put in a position to help their own communities, they could do it." In the long run many of the most basic problems came down to whether they should "get local people to do something, or get professionals to come in and do it for you. We are too poor to hire professionals everywhere, all the time."

After thinking it through, they decided the first issue was the mothers' ability to mix the solution.

Directions that called for using a teaspoon would be no help; the village people don't have or use teaspoons routinely. Sugar was to be used, but which sugar? Refined white sugar was not commonly available and was expensive. What the villagers more often had was *gur*, a brown sugar made from local cane or date juice. Analysis soon showed that *gur* was actually better than refined sugar because it often contained small amounts of potassium and bicarbonate—which were ingredients in the official oral rehydration solution.

So Abed started from scratch, in his own kitchen, with ingredients from the street. He took local salt, *lobon*, *gur*, and a tin cup common in the villages, a *seer*. After Abed and his wife cooked up dozens of batches of differing measures, they were sent to the Cholera Research

Laboratory. The homemade concoction that proved closest to the official WHO formula was the following: a pinch of salt (in Bangladesh, it's a three-finger pinch using the index finger, middle finger, and thumb), two small scoops of *gur*, and half a *seer* of water. Later it was modified slightly in the field, because women use their hollowed palms to measure scoops. One "fist" was about two scoops.

After much more work, the formula finally became a simple chant: "a pinch, a fist, and half a *seer*." The mixture was dubbed "*lobon-gur* solution" and the first great trial of the fundamental question—could illiterate mothers be taught to make and use *lobon-gur* successfully?— began in Sulla, Bangladesh, in February 1979.

BRAC carefully selected teachers (the first two were young village women, Hemlata Sarkar and Shwapna Bowmick), wrote and tested a teaching method several times, and only gradually spread the experiment from Sulla to other villages. Routinely, they took samples from the solutions made by mothers and sent them to the Cholera Research Laboratory for analysis.

Doctors in Bangladesh felt their turf was the treatment of human illness and that BRAC's experiments were now starting to invade that territory. One official from the World Health Organization rushed to Bangladesh to try to get the government to greatly expand its anti-diarrhea program to head off BRAC. But that program was poorly planned and did not take into account the scale and difficulties of the problem.

BRAC went ahead, and over the next year young women trainers in groups of six moved through 662 villages, a few weeks in each village, attempting to train 58,000 mothers in the new treatment method.

One thing distinctive about this project when compared to many "development" projects over the years is that it was carried out entirely locally, by people who had become deadly serious about making it work. So the many mistakes and repeated trouble in this or that part of the program were confronted, not ignored. That doing and redoing turned out to be the most difficult part. After the first thirty thousand women were trained, and their competence had been checked and rechecked by visits from monitors, Abed said, they reached a first plateau. It was thrilling to have built the project up so far, especially as it was under fire even as it carried on.

"This was our first opportunity to scale-up programs from small areas to the whole nation," he said. "When we got done teaching the first thirty thousand mothers, we went back to check how we had succeeded. But we found that of all the women who had been taught the method, only six percent were using it when their children became sick. I was very disappointed. Disheartened. Why should we be going from house to house teaching women to do this if then they are not going to use it?"

Abed and the other leaders of BRAC believed in it. It was technically sound and medically potent, truly lifesaving. "We decided there must be something wrong with our teaching. The commitment we had was not being transmitted, somehow."

They heard of one case when a mother with a very sick baby was visited by a young BRAC worker. The worker quickly suggested running down to the medicine shop for some diarrhea medicine, saying, "It will be quicker."

Abed, talking about it now, looks down at his desk. "So we found out that some of our workers didn't believe in what they were teaching. They thought our homemade solution was crude, second-rate."

Abed realized their earlier explanations had been too sketchy and had not caught the imaginations of their workers. So he rounded up all three hundred workers of the time and started from the beginning, explaining why this solution was lifesaving and that anything else, short of intensive hospital treatment, could be deadly. They explained the infections that cause diarrhea and the reaction of the bowel; they gave details of why sugar and salt were crucial. They talked about the number of deaths of children in the villages in which they were working.

"Once workers became convinced this was the best therapy, their whole attitude changed, their behavior changed. They became committed," he said.

In all BRAC work, that is now a vital test of whether a project will succeed or fail. Do the workers understand it? Are they excited, committed?

When they went back a little while later to check again, "we found things had improved a little—now twenty-one percent of mothers were using the method. But again, we were not very happy."

There was another element they hadn't considered enough. They decided to bring in some anthropologists to talk to the mothers and other villagers about BRAC and diarrhea and their lives in general.

"We found that the women were not the only ones we had to convince. They were not the sole decision makers in the house or in the village," he said. There were the husbands and brothers, who would say, "Don't use that cheap method, I don't trust it." And there were the local traditional healers who advised against using the BRAC method. So they added to their effort visits to the men in the villages, talks in the marketplace, and later added even radio advertising.

This round of effort pushed the rate of usage up over 50 percent, Abed said. Still not enough.

On further probing they found some of the workers were doing their teaching in too rote a fashion when they were tired, and some even cheated, skipping the teaching and mixing up solution themselves and sending for tests as if the mothers had made it. So a further round of fixes went in. They set up monitoring and paid the rehydration teachers not on the basis of houses covered, or sessions with mothers, but on the basis of a sampling of the actual performance of the mothers. For each mother who could answer questions and make an effective *lobon-gur* solution, the worker would get paid a certain amount. For each mother who was taught but did not perform well, the BRAC workers earned less.

And on it went. "The commitment grew, and the teachers began to get more creative and involved," Abed said. Eventually they were able to get the quality of teaching up and routinely get mothers to make the solution right over 98 percent of the time. The rate of death from diarrhea began to drop across the nation.

"I have seen a lot of bad development projects," Abed said. "It is not that the people doing them are not sincere. They are. But in many cases, whether they come from outside the country or from inside, they expect to work a project for three years, do the best they can, and then go on to something else.

"But in BRAC we were there for the long haul. We were committed to building the country forever. We wanted to make sure things really change. We were totally results-oriented from the beginning. That made quite a lot of difference."

The project took ten years, but by the time it was over it was firmly rooted in the national psyche. Entrepreneurs soon began to take advantage of it, and started importing and selling packets of rehydration salts throughout the nation and in all the village medicine shops. Mothers could now make their own or, if they could afford it, buy the salts and work from there. The treatments of deadly diarrhea were now in their hands. The whole BRAC project from 1979 to 1990 cost about $9.3 million.

By 1990, the word had spread, and oral rehydration was being used in dozens of countries around the world. In 1991, one of the worst epidemics of cholera since the nineteenth century struck South America and Mexico. But the usual rate of death—one-third to one-half—did not materialize. In this epidemic millions of packets of salts were flown in and put in the hands of local medical people and villagers. The death rate when the epidemic died down proved to be nearer 1 percent than 50 percent. The transmission of Bangladesh's success was, in fact, another kind of globalization.

In the end the object is really to give the people in the villages some mental and physical skills so they can do the work on their own, in their own villages.

During the years of scaling up the diarrheal disease treatment, BRAC also began its project to start village schools. Many girls in the villages were never sent to school, or soon dropped out because the work seemed irrelevant (mostly to parents) to their daily chores at home. So BRAC decided to take the village dropouts, about 70 percent of them girls, and offer a few hours of instruction per day. This is Bangladesh, the country with the densest population, so teaching just dropouts became a large task. Now BRAC has thirty-four thousand schools, which is said to be the largest private school network in the world. Each school is a single room with jute mats, chalk slates, and a few books for thirty students. Across Bangladesh, there are now 1 million students in the schools, and over the last couple of decades the system has graduated 2.8 million children; 92 percent of them have gone on to secondary school. The cost of the whole system is about eighteen dollars per pupil per year. To keep up the mental opportunities for the village girls after the primary years, BRAC added on libraries—there are now 873 libraries, 168 mobile libraries, and 8,800 discussion clubs for the village girls after they graduate.

BRAC was also among the first to create a "micro-finance" plan for the poor. It works as a series of village cooperative "banks." About twenty-five to thirty-five mothers in each village join the BRAC Village Organization, then with BRAC's help begin to make microloans. At this level, they take on only poor women who have no collateral and want very small loans—essentially those people commercial banks have no interest in. By 2004, the number of women in these Village Organizations was 4.7 million.

All the members are poor, and virtually all are women, by design. They give out loans, along with doing some other community duties. The average loan the women give to their neighbors is $117. It is to be paid back over a year, in weekly installments. This is enough money to buy a few chickens, or a milk cow, or to get a big patch of vegetables going for food and for resale. One woman bought her husband a rickshaw, which now is the family transportation business. The loans are not always used for burgeoning businesses; the women may buy a few chickens but not build up to a large chicken farm. But about 15 percent succeed in building the tiny loans into bigger things—a success rate said to be about the same for small business loans (tens to hundreds of thousands of dollars) in wealthy countries.

Though the women are poor, the organization is tidy, and the accounting careful: The repayment rate is above 98 percent and has remained steady at that rate for more than two decades. The total amount loaned so far to the villagers is more than $2.5 billion, and their current savings accounts total about $122 million.

It was as the programs for women and girls began to take off that fundamentalists began to notice BRAC and take it seriously. Some of the schools teaching village girls were burned down; the facilities lending to women were attacked; some called for the arrest of Abed. Eventually BRAC headquarters was bombed. But Bangladeshis condemned the actions and kept working with BRAC. This is interesting evidence of just what kind of work can successfully counter terrorism at the grassroots level.

"The reaction," said Abed, "confirmed our belief that we were on the right track."

Bill Gates Sr. once visited a BRAC village school and asked the girls in one class, "What do you want to be when you grow up?" Gates wrote later that one girl stood up and said, "I'm going to be a doctor." Not, "I want to be a doctor," but, "I am *going* to be a doctor." "I will never forget that moment," Gates wrote. "A little girl, daughter of poor, illiterate parents, sitting on a grass mat, over a dirt floor, in a one-room hut with a tin roof, telling me with total confidence: 'I am going to be a doctor.' I thought: this little one-room school house is changing the world."

During the hardest times, when BRAC was beginning, Abed now says that he would sometimes recite to himself a poem of the Bengali writer Rabindranath Tagore. When you go out to begin your journey, the poem begins, "if you call out to your friend to join you . . . and your friend upon hearing your call does not come along with you, then start to walk this path alone."

In recent years, visitors to BRAC have come away impressed to the point that they begin to say unlikely things. BRAC has been called "the greatest development group ever." It has been said to be "the world model for creating health and wealth in poor places." But there is really no model for the world; that is one of the things BRAC has proved. Model is the wrong word, the wrong idea. But its work has established some attitudes, some guiding ideas.

Abed and BRAC started with disaster relief, but soon enough the underlying truth became clear: The disaster was not a hurricane or a war; it was in the desperate poverty that had already existed and had gone on without useful aid year after year.

But now we know a few things about this state of affairs. We know that citizen organizations can be effective, not only in small programs but in very large ones. We know that villagers can be trained to do effective, lifesaving work. We know that continuous monitoring and reworking to achieve results is vital. And through it all, the workers must believe in what they are doing.

Abed himself says the changes began at least in part with the spirit of independence that reminded people here of Gandhi and Nehru in their grand quest, and that led to enthusiastic Bangladeshis who became determined to change life at the ground level. Some of them worked for BRAC, some worked for other groups. The government of Bangladesh, while often unable to lead the effort, cooperated and encouraged and partnered at key moments. This is nation building from the inside, but not without help from the outside.

The creation of BRAC took years, and the successes did not just fall naturally from goodwill and effort. But something was learned in BRAC and similar projects over the past three decades. This learning is, I suspect, the equal of any of the great technology and science discoveries of the past half century. In numbers of lives saved alone, even though the development work is just beginning, these discoveries may already be greater.

Now they must be applied.

In early 2005, in his Dhaka office, though Abed is nearly seventy he is talking about the future. A whole new "BRAC" has begun in Afghanistan, he says, and he has already told the minister of health that the program will cut infant mortality in half within five years in the district where they are working.

"When she heard that she said to me: 'Good luck!'" He laughs, draws on his pipe, and says immunization has been scaled up in all the districts where they are working. Now, he says, the government has asked him to expand to more districts.

Isn't that risky? Will you prove it out in the few districts first or will you go big so soon?

"Go big!" he says, and smiles. "We can't wait around with the children dying; we've got to try." Now, he says, he is sending teams to some African countries to consider getting BRAC-like groups started there as well.

Abed ends by quoting an old BRAC saying. "'Small is beautiful,'" he says, "'but big is necessary.'"

2

Forty-nine Thousand Grandmothers

Saving Nepal's Children

The young woman stops what she is doing. Even late in the afternoon, the light is strong here in Sarlahi, Nepal, in the emerald green rice fields of the Ganges river plain. But each afternoon about this time, just as the sky begins to cool, Yamuna Sharma hastens home, because she knows what is coming.

At dusk every evening she goes blind. It will not pass until dawn.

She is wearing a bright yellow sari, and she moves quickly toward her mud-brick home. The huts here are close together, with wet paths between them only wide enough for an ox pulling a small cart to get by. Some huts are one room, some two, and they house eight or ten family members. The kitchen is outside: a stool next to a fireplace. There is no plumbing.

This is the southern part of Nepal—the flat, rich tableland set before the Himalayas. It can get steamy and hot here, routinely over 100°F in the summer. And then there are the monsoons, an annual but unpredictable wave of storms needed to replenish the water in the rice paddies.

On this August evening there is something different in the village. People from the Nepali National Vitamin A Program will be visiting Yamuna Sharma, bringing some visitors from Europe and America. They have heard from workers in the area that Yamuna has gone night-blind, and they want to talk to her about the condition. It used to be a very common problem here; the midwives all know it, as it often used to come during pregnancy. But now it is rare.

They are investigating a project that has become famous among those who deliver aid to developing countries, who work in the bad spots of the world. This place and the nutrition program here are famous for two reasons. First, because research here proved one of the most surprising propositions of the last fifty years of medicine. Second, because the project that was built on that surprising research is among the simplest and most cost-effective ways to save lives ever devised. If there could be a model for the world of how to deliver a life-saving intervention cheaply, this is it.

As the visitors arrive at Yamuna's hut, she settles in near her front door. Yamuna squats with her legs in front of her, and she wraps them with her skinny arms. She is nervous about talking without her husband present. Soon a little knot of children and other villagers settles near to eavesdrop on the odd visit. They seem to be entertained by this village version of a TV special.

Yamuna is pregnant with her second child, but this time she has encountered this peculiar disorder. From time to time as she speaks softly, she pulls her head scarf across her face to hide.

But she will be okay; she's within the small circle of safety that is the hut. Each day the world around her dims to black. We talk to her as her vision slips away. She is saying that sometimes she stumbles. She has tried to serve dinner, but can't do it, to her shame. She once dumped rice on the table instead of on a plate. At night she must be led about or sit by herself in a corner.

She talks quietly about her "weakness," as she calls it. She says she sometimes awakes before it is light, lying anxious, waiting for the curse to be lifted. Night blindness is not the worst problem of life here. But it is certainly the source of trouble in families, as women with it can do no work after dusk, though their duties to provide meals and clean the house are plain. For affected children it is another kind of affliction, for early night is their best chance to be free to play in the darkened streets with friends and sibs. Instead of running free, they soon became the object of fun and sometimes meanness.

When the visitors are finished chatting, Yamuna is offered a dose of vitamin A in a capsule. After explanations, she accepts. By the next night, her night blindness is gone.

Not long ago, it was discovered, much to the surprise of nutritionists and doctors, that night blindness was not just a problem on its own. It is a flag marking the occurrence of something far worse.

The story of this discovery is one of the better tales in modern public medicine. It is now estimated that this little finding, and the interventions which followed, save about one million lives—mostly children and pregnant women—every year. And as the work spreads, the number is expected to rise. In the middle of some of the most difficult places and hardest lives, it has brought some relief even where there is no doctor and no nearby clinic.

The story of vitamin A in developing countries has also become part of something bigger—a new approach to bringing vital services to people in developing countries, cheaply and through their own efforts. The approach does not have one name or an identifiable set of adherents; rather, it is emerging across disciplines everywhere at once. It has affected everyone, from the economists in international banks to the local health posts in the toughest places in the world. It is the result of years of work in poor countries, both by trial and error and by rigorous academic research.

For many years, conservatives have argued that aid to poor countries is, as Senator Jesse Helms once said, "money poured down a rat hole." But sentiments have begun to shift on that side of the aisle. (Senator Helms himself on his retirement repented some of his stubbornness and testified that he was ashamed that he had done so little to help the children of other nations, suggesting that America give an additional $500 million gift to fight AIDS in Africa.)

One official sign of the change came when Andrew Natsios, President Bush's chief of the key U.S. Agency for International Development, spoke before the Heritage Foundation in May 2002. Heritage is one of the conservative groups that has most strongly criticized foreign aid. Heritage's position, as characterized by the *Foreign Service Journal*, had been, "Foreign aid doesn't work. Trade, not aid, works. U.S. dollars are going down a rat hole. Corrupt foreign elites grow fat off American aid." Natsios told those gathered at the Heritage meeting that President Bush had committed his administration to another approach. The president himself had just pledged an increase in foreign aid from $10 billion to $15 billion a year over the following three budget years. Not that the administration wanted to renew old-style aid, Natsios said, but that "smart aid" was the new way forward. He pointed out that in East Asia foreign assistance had been vital to the creation of the Asian Tigers—Korea, Thailand, and Malaysia. "Private domestic investment and rapidly growing human capital were the principal engines of growth," he said. The plan is to give more aid, but make sure it goes to aid programs that can prove they are effective.

While such political pull-and-tug is happening at the high levels of policy, so it is also happening at the lowest levels—on the ground in developing countries. The vitamin A program is one of a number of projects that are examples of what can have a real, measurable impact on health. Key features of it are that it is backed by data proving its effectiveness, and while it is carried out with the help of the Nepalese government, the money supporting the program goes directly to the groups running the program, not to the government treasury. Though experts don't want to call this kind of targeted, evidence-based program a "magic bullet," they are hopeful that it offers at least one good model that can be used to avoid the old canards of corruption and aid "rat holes."

The story of the building of this project, from lab research to life-saving moments, began with a surprise in Java, then moved to Nepal, where forty-nine thousand grandmothers began to make use of the new knowledge.

Alfred Sommer is a medical researcher with both a great interest in human vision and a significant case of wanderlust.

He is a lanky fellow, thin and trim, with his hair slicked back, old-fashioned eyeglasses, and conservative dress. He is now the dean of one of the top schools of public health in the world—Johns Hopkins Bloomberg School of Public Health. In 1970 he was a thirty-year-old doctor in search of a medical and intellectual adventure. He wasn't much interested in working in a clinic. Instead, he went to the Centers for Disease Control, where he became one of the elite corps called the Epidemic Intelligence Service. These are the disease detectives who investigate new outbreaks, from Ebola fever in the Congo to Legionnaire's disease in Philadelphia. When his tour with the CDC was up, he headed out to Asia.

In his first large investigation he set up camp in a village in Indonesia to interview and give medical exams to all the children in the six villages surrounding West Java; there were forty-six hundred children and their families all told. He wanted to find out just how widespread blindness caused by vitamin A deficiency was and what might be done about it.

The condition is called xerophthalmia, or night blindness. It comes from a shortage of vitamin A in the body, because the rods of the eye—the part that senses low levels of light—depend on a supply of it to operate. People have noticed the symptom for thousands of years, and in several languages it is called "chicken eyes," because chickens can't see in the dark. When the shortage of vitamin A gets severe in humans it leads to other symptoms besides night blindness: dry eyes and small white ulcers on the skin of the eye called Bitot's spots. As the disease progresses the wall of the eye weakens, sores can develop, and a total collapse of the eye and permanent blindness results. Because of infection and other complications, the condition can sometimes be fatal.

Sommer and his team of thirteen, including two doctors, two nurses, a nutritionist, and eight other aides, gave general medical exams as well as eye exams to the children in the Java villages every three months. As he found, the relationship of a visiting scientist to the people under study is symbiotic, like the egrets that perch on a hippo's back plucking insects. The doctors treat some problems the children have, or send them to a clinic; what the doctors get in return is data, the vital scientific essence that makes knowledge and careers.

His first round of work was finished in 1981, and with it the world had its first real estimate of how much nutrition-caused blindness there is. Sommer found that in Indonesia alone there were sixty thousand cases per year. Extrapolating to Asian countries with similar populations—India, Bangladesh, and the Philippines—he wrote that these four nations produce five hundred thousand cases per year, several times the previous estimates.

After publishing the new information Sommer went back to Baltimore, to his small office at the Johns Hopkins public health school. It was Christmas vacation time in 1982 when he started to write another paper from the data he had collected. He was hoping to explain what it was that made the children low in vitamin A. Severe diarrhea, he speculated, might flush a good deal of nutrition, and vitamins, from their systems.

But as he searched for the night-blind children in the data sheets, he kept coming up blank. They had started the study, but they were missing at the end. Eventually the reason became clear: They had died.

Why? It did not take long before he realized he had got it exactly backward. It was not that vitamin A shortages came after diarrhea; it was that diarrhea came after vitamin A shortage. It could be that the low vitamin A was *bringing on* more infection, not *resulting* from it. As he added up the numbers it became plain that more than a third of all the night-blind children died early. Those without it remained much healthier.

Somehow, a low level of vitamin A might be making children vulnerable to infection and death.

Among the one-year-olds in the villages they found about eight out of every thousand had died. But when they asked after the children with night blindness, twelve times as many had died—one hundred per thousand—just since their visit three months before.

He also could see that the risk of death increased directly in proportion to how low the children's vitamin A was. If they had mild night blindness, their risk of death was about triple that of children with normal vision. If they had developed another form of vitamin A deficiency, Bitot's spots, their risk of death was four times normal. And if they had signs of both, their risk of death was almost nine times normal.

He then looked to see what the children were dying of. There was little surprise there—pneumonia and diarrhea, the usual killers of children in poor countries in Asia. It seemed as if vitamin A must be needed to defend against infections.

Sommer went to the library. He looked up the history of the vitamin; to his surprise, he found that over the years other researchers had reported just the kind of thing he was seeing—vitamins as a factor in preventing infection. But the knowledge somehow had been lost. Not long after Sommer's early-twentieth-century predecessor at Johns

Hopkins Elmer McCollum and colleagues discovered vitamin A, their research had also demonstrated its uses.

In those days the science of nutrition was just beginning, and McCollum, on farms in Wisconsin, had done the simple and obvious experiments to find out what was needed in diets. He fed animals diets that began with the simplest things, for example, rice alone. That was clearly deficient; rats lost their fur and couldn't survive on it. Gradually, he isolated key ingredients in a healthy diet that had not been that obvious.

It had been assumed that meat was a natural part of a man's diet. The value of vegetables was not as clear. And, as it turned out, there were a list of "hidden" ingredients that humans needed to have in small amounts in their diet; they were dubbed "vitamins," and named in the order that McCollum and others found them, with A first. If humans ate an animal-based diet, including meat and liver and so on, all the essential ingredients and the hidden ingredients were present; it made sense that humans who had evolved as hunter-gatherers would have a diet based on the ingredients animals had in their bodies.

But diets had changed over the millennia, and things got out of proportion. Meat at one time was part of the diet, but so were the berries, nuts, and leaves that humans gathered. Between 1913 and the mid-1930s researchers found that vitamins, including A, could be taken in from both animal parts and fruits and vegetables.

McCollum tried various experiments on animals. In one series, he fed animals a diet which had a single source of fat. He found that lard, almond oil, and olive oil as the sole sources were defective, leading to loss of vision and hair, skin problems, and sometimes death. But rats given butter, cod liver oil, or egg yolk as the sole source remained largely healthy. He isolated the key difference between the fats that worked and those that didn't: It was the presence of vitamin A.

Campaigns for healthy eating, and bringing back the neglected parts of the human diet, grew out of his work, along with campaigns to supplement the diet with syrups or pills of vitamins.

It was eventually called "vitamania," as writer Scott Shane had noted. The sales of vitamins went up more than tenfold between the 1930s and 1940s. By 1951, *Time* magazine was calling McCollum "Dr. Vitamin" and saying, "He has done more than any other man to put vitamins back in the nation's bread and milk, to put fruit on American breakfast tables, fresh vegetables and salad greens in the daily diet."

What was learned in the first half of the twentieth century but eventually forgotten was that with vitamin A the subject is not vision, but skin. It is skin that needs vitamin A—the lining of the mouth, the eye, the lungs, and the whole digestive system all need vitamin A. In the lungs and gut, without vitamin A the cilia and mucus cells in the skin die off and cannot snare and carry off invaders. For the children of Indonesia, where the environment is laden with microbial hazards, the lack of vitamin A was impairing one of their key defenses, the skin cells that kept out germs.

Sommer found papers from the 1920s and 1930s that showed vitamin A could help stop infection. In addition to pneumonia and diarrhea, Sommer found that measles became a killer of children in Africa and elsewhere because it depleted the system of vitamin A, leaving the sick children open to new infections. Thus, the death rate from measles was much higher than the viral infection itself warranted. In a study in Tanzania Sommer and his colleagues were able to cut the death rate from measles in half. But as he reported this finding later, he noted with chagrin that almost an identical study had been done—with the same results—in a London hospital in 1932.

Sommer was determined that the importance of vitamin A should not be forgotten again.

He and his colleagues published a paper announcing the new findings on vitamin A in the fall of 1983 in the British medical journal *The Lancet*. Alongside the finding was a critical commentary by another scientist. The latter ran under the heading: "Too Good to Be True."

Fair enough. It did seem improbable. There are so many things wrong with the lives of poor children in developing countries; it seemed unlikely that one identifiable and fixable problem could account for a third of the deaths among children.

The reaction to the article overall was resounding silence. Sommer was not sure what to do, how to begin arguing with the wall of stone disbelief he was facing. A colleague told him that if he believed it, there was only one way to make other doctors believe it: Bury them in data. Do the study again, and again, with full controls and care, in different places, until the sheer mass of data became impossible to ignore.

And so he did.

He began a large-scale study in the Philippines in the summer of 1983, but soon became the target of anti-American rebels and the study had to be shut down. He lost more than a year of work but changed venues and began a large study among the children of 450 villages in Sumatra. In this study, 25,939 children were examined, and those with night blindness were immediately treated and left out of the study. But among those with no sign of low vitamin A, half were given vitamin A supplements twice during the next year, and half served as controls. All the children were examined again at the end of the study, and supplements were provided.

During the year of study, the death rate for children who got the vitamin drops was cut by more than one-third.

This time, the reaction when the study was published was not silence. This time, Sommer says, "There were howls. The knives came out." He pauses and adds, more philosophically, that Rudolf Virchow, the pioneer of public medicine in nineteenth-century Germany, said that the stages of acceptance of an extraordinary result in science are like the stages of grief. First there is disbelief. Then there is anger. Finally, the critics say we knew it all along; it's obvious.

The huge number of children in the study made it very strong, but critics still had difficulty accepting the idea. Criticism focused on the fact that the study contained no placebo controls. The Indonesian government wouldn't allow a study in which fake medicine was given intentionally, so the plan instead introduced a vitamin A campaign, and compared those who got vitamin A in the first year with those who had not gotten it yet.

Critics pointed out that with such a design it was possible that those getting the vitamin A drops might also have benefited from the additional attention and care brought when the researchers showed up in their villages. Maybe it wasn't the vitamin; maybe it was that villagers started bringing their children to the local clinic more often. Worse, a study in India had failed to find the magical effect of vitamin A.

Thus, still another huge study was planned, this time in Nepal. This would be the deciding test.

The study began in September 1989, in the rice-growing southern district of Sarlahi. It was put there because the regional is so similar to large parts of India, Bangladesh, and other regions of Asia—if the results were good, they should be applicable elsewhere. The study included 28,630 children and was intended to run for two years. But after one year, when the data was analyzed, the effect of vitamin A was so powerful that it would have been unethical to continue. The study was stopped, and vitamin A given to all the children. The study found, once again, that the death rate was 30 percent lower in the children getting the drops. Among the older children, five and six years old, the effect was even stronger—a 50 percent drop in the death rate.

The paper which followed concluded, "Thus, periodic Vitamin A delivery in the community can greatly reduce child mortality in developing countries." The paper also estimated that if the vitamin was given routinely to preschool children about 15,000 deaths a year could be avoided in Nepal alone, and about one million deaths in South Asia prevented each year.

Sommer wrote, "Too often we expect that complicated issues require complicated solutions; too often we follow the obvious and ignore or reject the unexpected." Some health officials still refused to believe the implication of the studies: Two cents worth of vitamin A could have a profound impact on the survival of children around the world.

By the end of 1992, however, researchers had been at work and produced at least eight large studies of vitamin A in five countries. In all but one the effect was very large and consistent—about a third of childhood deaths could be avoided if the right amount of vitamin A was given.

Forcing knowledge can be hard; it took from 1913 to about 1992 for nutritionists and doctors to accept the fundamentals of vitamin A. But in the end, that may have been the easy part.

The next step was to take those findings and apply them in the most troublesome places in the world. In 1992, the World Health Organization held a meeting in Bellagio, Italy, where twenty-five of the top nutrition researchers from around the world met to set out the final consensus: Vitamin A works, and in addition, it can be delivered cheaply. An economic analysis done by the World Bank showed that vitamin A treatment would be among the most cost-effective treatments ever devised. For about fifty cents, including the vitamin and the cost of delivery, death could be cut substantially. The bank estimated that for every dollar spent on vitamin A treatment, about one hundred dollars would be returned to society in the form of work and productivity.

The government of Nepal, having hosted the crucial test of vitamin A, was ready to go ahead and deliver it to its children. At least in theory. In practice, such delivery would be very hard to set up and maintain.

To begin with, Nepal had a tiny national health budget that was already tied up in maintaining small health clinics in districts around the country. Unfortunately, as in many places, this system was top-heavy with administrators and disappointingly unresponsive to citizens at the lowest level. As in many places people largely avoided clinics when they could, because they often had to walk many kilometers to reach them, had to wait in long queues when they arrived, and in the end felt they didn't get much for their trouble. The idea of visiting the clinic often throughout the year was unthinkable for many. If the delivery of vitamin A were simply added to the work of the little clinics in villages across the country, the result could easily be failure. How would the people learn how important it was? Would they believe it? Would they come out an extra two or three times a year? What if they were charged for such visits, as Western economists were insisting?

The math alone made a vitamin A program hard to imagine: If workers were paid only a small amount, 100 rupees to deliver doses of vitamin A in their communities, this alone would amount to 5 million rupees, not counting the supplies and other things needed to get the work done.

This is the problem of everyday life in the developing world: It is hard to make things work, and every possibility is met with two problems.

The work in Nepal sprang from the work of some of the researchers in Sommer's school, including Keith West and Steve LeClerq. The U.S. Agency for International Development was convinced to keep funding up after the research was done and put it into the practical delivery program. In the end, a large part of the responsibility for building a vitamin A program in Nepal fell to a young local man, Ram Shrestha, who hailed from the villages in which the research had been carried out.

Nepal has had some of the worst poverty and the highest rates of child death in the world. Nearly one of three children born in the rural areas did not survive to their fifth birthday. Outside of a few cities, the people of the nation are living in conditions very like those of two hundred years ago.

It is possible to parachute in aid and modern health care for some people, for limited periods of time. This has been done in most every country of the developing world, more than once. Some of the flown-in programs have been successful and inspiring; some have failed. These efforts, both good and bad, have been treated largely as charity work. Healers and experts came to the country, carried out their good works for a few months or years. There had been little pressure to consider this kind of missionary-style work as something that should be built into lasting local institutions that solved local problems. The problems of poverty and suffering in the developing world were counted as simply too enormous to solve, and difficult enough to address even for short periods in limited locales. All projects were for the better, as long as some people were helped.

These ways of thinking were interrupted by the 1990s. As in the nineteenth century, the growth of global trade has like a bulldozer driven attitudes and realities ahead of it as it cleared ground for more profitable, open trade. The need for security in each region of the globe has become more urgent. New ways of collecting and understanding information about how societies work has begun to push aside traditional, clumsy economic models. The words "sustainable" and "accountable" and "transparent" have begun to express a different way of thinking about how one nation helps another. The old and new thinking are still entangled; both are used, and there is nothing that will guarantee that the best solutions are reached, or that old-fashioned power and greed will be overcome as globalization moves ahead. But there is a good chance.

From each country, and with each new attempt to push back poverty and promote development, there are now stories of success that can point the way to new, workable approaches.

The creation of the new ways has often come from the people at work in the countries, not from economists or theorists elsewhere. It is most often people trying to get a job done who have begun to understand and deliver what is needed.

In Nepal, after the vitamin A experiments were complete, the problems were posed there. We can reduce the death rate in children dramatically, even where the poverty is extreme and medical assistance is nearly absent. But how? Do we try to reenergize the government health posts? Do we build a separate army of nongovernmental workers to deliver several key services? Do we find local people and turn over the tasks to them?

In Nepal, the poor fellow who was confronted with the task of creating a system to deliver vitamin A to the whole population was Ram Shrestha, chemist and nutrition worker from Saptari in southern Nepal. With the blessing of government, a small packet of funds, and little else, he began to create a new nongovernmental organization called the Nepal Technical Assistance Group.

He is a small, round man with a characteristic Nepali grin. Shrestha is the fourth of seven children born in a farming village, and he says he was very lucky to be a middle child. In the cultures of

Nepal, the eldest and the youngest have a great burden of duties, cere-monial and practical. There is relatively little expected of the middle children in the way of careers. "I could do anything," he says. "And I did."

He grew up speaking the local dialects of Nepali, but because much of the culture is still in the shadow of India, Hindi was the lan-guage of education and advancement, and he learned that as well. But when he excelled in the local school and his father wanted him to learn science or medicine, at age fifteen he was sent to the nearest center of learning, in Kathmandu.

When he first arrived in the city he was frightened, because as he stepped outside the home where he was staying, what he gazed upon were buildings back to back and pavement side to side, with no grass, little sky.

As he puts it, "When I looked out, there was nothing! How could people be here?" To find his way around he began by identifying a tower near the house and memorizing the way from the tower to home. Then, his job was to spot the tower, go to it, and follow the fa-miliar path home.

After getting a basic college degree, he didn't have the money or the high grades to earn a full scholarship, so he found a job in what came naturally to him—language. He worked for the Peace Corps, teaching young Americans to speak Nepali. As a second job, he signed up to work in a research lab run by Johns Hopkins. His job was to watch monkeys behave and to record, moment by moment, what they did.

"That taught me about how to observe," he says. "And how to dis-cipline myself." He had to be continuously alert for hours at a time, and had to follow the animals' lead, resting when they rested, making notes when they were active, always ready for sudden outbreaks of fighting.

When his work on this project was finished, he kept looking for opportunities to study; one came along when a local university offered a program in what was called "development services." After the classroom work each student was sent to a distant village to teach in school and lead a development project.

He was sent first to the Jajarkot district in the west, and from there traveled from place to place. He learned at times to live off the land, so to speak.

"Wherever I traveled, I took aspirin with me," he says. Armed with it, he could knock on any door in search of a meal. After chatting up someone, "you just ask, does anyone have stomach pain, a headache? You will find, definitely, they have some pains. Or if not them, their grandmothers. So you can then say, Ahh, I have medicine for you." They were unfamiliar with medicine, for the most part, so when their pains subsided, their relief was great enough to produce an invitation to dinner.

He also learned people-marshaling skills. In one village, a new hillside footpath was needed between a village and the nearby clinic. At first, he tried to recruit parents, who said they were too busy and too tired. Few answered the call. But soon, Ram began to use his authority at school. He recruited the children to recruit their families, offering them school credit for help and school demerits if they failed. The families showed up with their hoes and made quick work of the new path.

After his experiences in the villages, he returned to school to earn a master's degree in chemistry. But when he began looking for work, he wanted something that would entail working with the public, like the Peace Corps or public health projects. After scouring the catalogs of international studies and filling out piles of applications, what turned up was a course in international nutrition offered by Tufts University in Massachusetts.

He got back to Nepal in 1991, just as plans were being made to build the vitamin A program. He took up the job of finding and training workers to carry it out.

First, he spent time going from place to place, talking to those working in the new program. "I wanted to understand how it was working and not working," he says.

Programs had come through, and people in the villages had come forward to work. They were called volunteers, but actually they were paid. When polio workers were needed, they were paid. The understanding was that when the government or foreigners had projects they wanted done, they came and paid people to do them. This seemed reasonable, but there was not enough money, and it raised other problems as well.

Ram began to feel that if anything were to get done the issue should not be about money, but about motivation. The approach had been backward.

The object was to save the lives of children in the villages. So how had it become an intervention from *outside*? How was it that the parents of the children themselves did not feel part of it? There was reluctance to do the job, and suspicion between the people and the outsiders.

So when Ram began to recruit people to work in giving out vitamin A, he did not start by talking about the virtues of the vitamin. He began by going from village to village asking, What are the biggest problems in this village?

In the meetings, he asked villagers to talk about what was killing the children—diarrhea, malnutrition, and measles. He raised the question of whether there were some things that the village people could do to stop the constant waves of sickness. If there were one or two things that made a great difference, he asked the villagers, would you be willing to do them?

He spoke of the experience in Sarlahi and the vitamin A experiment. He talked about the children of Sarlahi. They are like our children, he said. They are poor; there is no sanitation, not enough food. The people there gave their children capsules with vitamin A, and where ten had died before, now three or four were saved. So is this worth doing here?

When villagers see the chance this way, as a local project, they want to get the capsules, Ram says. He told them that the capsules were available, and they could be brought to the village, but the villagers would have to create a reliable way to get them to all the children. Name a person or two in your neighborhood who will receive them and learn how to give them, he suggested. Then, on two days a year, the capsules will be there and you must get the children over to her house, or to the schoolyard. The capsules will be dropped into the mouths of the children then and there. "Can you do this?" he asked.

"I tried to say, but very softly so I would not lose my job, that this is not really a government program. This is your program. If you want it, you can do it. But if you just rely on government, this won't happen," Ram says.

With those who were to be the village distributors, a little more work was needed. They needed to get some training about how to store and use the capsules, how to keep track of the children who had gotten them and the ones who hadn't. They had to help get the word out about which day was the day to come get the capsule.

This project would have to be built on motives other than money. The love of their children, of course, was the vital starting point. But Ram felt more was needed. Delivering capsules was worthwhile for everyone in the village, so it followed that those doing the work should get some acknowledgment. He devised ways to get some recognition for those who volunteered.

When he first arrived in some of the districts from Kathmandu, he visited the district leader or ward chief.

He would pay his respects, and then ask if he knew the local volunteer who was going to be part of the big new program. The district leader would say no, but I can find her.

"I would then go out with them in the jeep, from place to place asking where the volunteer lived," he says. He knew where she lived, but he didn't let on. "It was better that the district chief was seen to be asking for her. Then the leader would visit the home," he says. And afterward, when there were occasional meetings about the vitamin A distribution, problems or strategies, Ram would make sure some of the meetings were in the homes of the volunteers, so that the officials came to the volunteers and not the other way around.

He determined at one point to print a cheap calendar so the

volunteers could keep track of the dates by which each task had to be done. "I put their pictures on it. So for at least thirty days, everyone would look at this one and that one," he says. When the donors paying for the vitamin A wanted to use radio advertising to announce the vitamin A days, they suggested using Bollywood stars. Ram said, No, we will use my volunteers to tell them.

He also gave the volunteers dark green canvas shoulder bags to use. "They were nothing. You have to add value," he says, and told the story of how he established the shoulder bag as the badge of the volunteer.

He went out to a market looking for a victim—someone carrying the green bag who shouldn't be. He spotted a man, and pulled up in his official vehicle and stopped him.

"Where did you get this bag?"

The man began to panic as if he was accused of theft. "This is my wife's bag . . ."

"No, this is a volunteer's bag. This is not your bag. So why are you carrying this?"

"My wife is a volunteer . . ."

"But it is her bag, not yours. Have you done anything for her? Have you distributed the vitamin A capsules? No."

The scene quickly turned into a ruckus, the shouting began, and eventually the police came. Ram had made his point clear: This is her bag, and if you carry it, you owe her. You cannot just have the bag.

By the next day the story had made the rounds and its point with the village.

While there is little money in the vitamin A program, there are a few organizers who have offices and vehicles. To press home his point, Ram instructed all those moving about in vehicles to stop whenever they saw a woman with the green bag. If they were going the same way, they would offer a lift, a valuable commodity in the villages. But if they were going the other way, they would promise to look out for them next time.

"What happened then? If the volunteer has to walk anywhere, the first thing they remember is to bring the bag, hoping someone will give them a lift," he says.

When visitors came to an area, they were brought to the volunteers' homes and asked to carry a green bag for a while. Ram wanted to make it clear to all that the visiting celebrity was there to visit the vitamin A volunteers.

Other programs had begun with requirements: You must be married, have children, have some ability to read, have some free time. But this program was to be carried out in every village in Nepal. There were just not enough women with energy, literacy, and free time. For this project, Ram targeted the greatest natural resource in the villages— the grandmothers.

He was told that it would not work; these village women were not up to the job. The were illiterate, of very low status, and suspicious of the officials from Kathmandu or the health department, and besides they might not be up to the work of traipsing house to house over many kilometers.

Literacy, Ram felt, was unimportant, and it would be a mistake to emphasize it. The women were unlettered but not stupid. They could quickly learn the value of the capsules and what was needed to deliver them. He also believed that the vitamins should not be delivered house to house. Rather, the villagers should come to get them. If they weren't willing to, he felt he would already have failed to get the basic message across. So a woman's ability to hike through the village wouldn't matter.

What the women soon found was that their new job as a volunteer earned them a place—and a bit of respect. At each turn Ram tried to reinforce the bits of respect and the perks available.

He has even carried on a little linguistic warfare of his own. In Nepali and Hindi, when a high status person is addressed, the speaker adds a syllable to their name. It would be Sharma-ji in Hindi or Sharma-jiu in Nepali. So he began to address his volunteers with the honorific attached. And in correspondence with suppliers and over- seers in the government, he would refer to his volunteers that way.

"This is very difficult for people," he says. "In the press releases or scripts we send to the radio, or in letters to the ministry, we would write 'Sharma-jiu.' They would always send it back, with it crossed out and corrected. I would retype and put the same thing again. It's a cold war, right? He doesn't say anything to me and I don't say anything to him. It has taken four years, but now people have started using it.

"You must find ways to give them status, respect in the village. We give them chances to speak in the district assembly. So they begin to feel the identity. He's a teacher. He's a doctor. I'm a volunteer."

And so it was that Ram Shrestha-jiu built a network of volunteers across Nepal. They are women, they are mostly older, they are mostly illiterate, but they can do the work.

There are now 49,000 such illiterate grandmothers giving vitamin capsules in Nepal twice each year. The project was built up over time. Of the 4 million children in Nepal, about 50,000 got vitamin A in the beginning, in 1993. The program reached only eight of the seventy-five districts in the country. But by 2004 more than 3.5 million children were routinely getting their vitamin, in all seventy-five districts. Coverage in each district ranged from about 91 percent to near 100 percent. The success was reflected in the crucial national numbers: In the 1980s, infant mortality in Nepal was 133 deaths for every 1,000 births. By 2002, the figure had dropped to 64, less than half.

It is now estimated that about 250,000 infant deaths are averted in Nepal each year by the vitamin program. Added to the program in 2000 was an effort to get vitamin A to pregnant women as well, since pregnancy severely depletes the body's reserves. As a measure of the success of that add-on program, the percentage of women who experience night blindness has dropped from 23 percent to 3 percent.

Year by year, the program was going so well that health officials couldn't resist beginning to add on other duties for the grandmothers who give vitamin A. They now also give deworming tablets to children to help stop infestations; they give iron supplements to mothers; and they have started a program to assure that families use iodized salt. Iodine in salt was first used to prevent the growths called goiters in developed countries, but as with vitamin A it was later found to have an even more vital effect—it prevents some kinds of mental retardation.

Ram says he is not sure how many different jobs can be loaded onto the backs of the grandmothers; he thinks if other villagers are willing to assist them, several more jobs may be taken on. But the biggest gain overall is that child deaths have dropped, and now it is the grandmothers getting the credit.

From his own experience Ram knows that motivation of any kind is, as he put it, "not stationary. It moves." In his own career he did prodigious amounts of work to earn a degree. But now it doesn't interest him much. "It's just paper." Then, a new kind of work came up that he didn't know how to do; he was curious; it became a challenge. That is, until he had been doing it for several years.

Other motivations needed to be built into the plan. He is now looking to add small in-kind payments for volunteers not unlike his "give-them-a-lift" initiative. For example, offering to give or subsidize some things that now must be paid for—perhaps schoolbooks, school uniforms. When children want to go on to higher levels of education, they must take exams, but the exams are not free. Perhaps volunteers' children might get the exams free.

One project he has started up that is now in about 10 percent of Nepal's districts is the "endowment fund." He asked the government in each district to set aside a small fund of fifty thousand rupees (about one thousand dollars). This money is not to be paid to the volunteers but to be put aside in an interest-bearing bank account. The interest from it is then periodically transferred to an account controlled by the women volunteers in that district (there are about nine per district). The women can then decide when and how to use the money.

"It is for their welfare. They can use it to have a party, to buy a sari. It's not much money. People asked if it was enough. I said it was not enough, but it was a start. At least they could have a cup of tea and a samosa. Without begging," he says.

He hopes eventually to expand the fund. Whenever an NGO comes in and wants some work done, the volunteers might meet with them and agree to do the work if the NGO would add another spot of money to the endowment fund. That way it might grow and become more useful.

But for the most part, Ram likes in-kind payments as a tool. The grandmother may be working in the vitamin program, but perhaps another member of the family is working as a volunteer in a forest conservation program, he says. "The benefit of that is that he can get firewood from the brush being cleared. You know, when someone brings home firewood, everyone is happy. But if he were to bring home money, they will fight. The husband wants to buy one thing, the son wants to buy another, and the wife wants a different thing."

There is a fear that this kind of volunteer network will ultimately fail. Also that it is fundamentally exploitive of the local people, getting substantial work from them for minimal compensation. But Ram argues that if the work they are doing fulfills their own needs, and people work to keep up the motivation, it may carry on for many years. It has already worked for five years.

One of the key lessons of vitamin A in Nepal, the same as in other successful health programs in poor areas, is that very simple interventions can yield large benefits.

This understanding is shaping up into new ways of thinking about health systems that give a different picture of these health systems in the developing world. Some things are best put into the hands of doctors, hospitals, and government clinics, as they stand now. But some things closer to home are out of their reach. (Not in theory, but in the way they have developed over the past three decades.)

To address these needs, money and expertise are needed, not to carry out programs, but rather to assist communities in building their own "grandmother" systems. It is clear that grandmother systems can deliver several interventions in neighborhoods. It is not known how many others can be added to the list.

The development of oral rehydration therapy to combat diarrhea in children discussed earlier is one of the early examples of community intervention. With the creation over the past century of new medicines and techniques, now is the time to simplify them and turn some of them over to ordinary people. Depending on highly educated people and elaborate health networks cannot work without some clever methods of spreading the knowledge and power.

In Nepal recently, another experiment showed that treatments once in the exclusive domain of doctors can now be farmed out to community workers. One case that proves the point in principle is an experiment carried out by researchers Nils Dulaire and Mary Taylor in Nepal beginning in 1986. Dulaire is now head of the Global Health Council in Washington, D.C.

Jumla is a little district in the northwestern corner of Nepal; it is surrounded by Himalayan peaks on three sides that rise above twenty thousand feet, and by a rough river on the fourth. From the main town in the district it is a five-day walk to reach the nearest tarred road out to the rest of the country. The only other way into the district is by fly-ing in to a dirt airstrip.

Even the bottoms of its valleys are above seven thousand feet, and so the farming life in this region is precarious. Warm season is short, the terrain rocky, and rain limited. There are chronic food shortages, and their death rates are among the highest in the world.

Life has changed little over the past several hundred years. Women do most of the work in the field, as well as make meals and raise chil-dren. But the women get little respect for all that; when their menses come they still are sent to sleep outside with the animals so that they do not contaminate the household.

Because the area is so remote and social and medical services are almost completely absent, researchers found it a pristine place to study. Their project was to deliver "affordable and sustainable inter-ventions . . . carried out using local villagers as health service delivery workers. It was recognized from the start that many well-intended community health programs have foundered because workers have been overwhelmed with too many activities to be digested and prop-erly conducted all at once; therefore, the Jumla workers would be trained to master the necessary tasks one limited set at a time."

They began with pneumonia as their target—it is the single largest killer of children in the world and in Jumla as well. They used a system newly accepted at the time that went by the typically awkward and opaque name "standard case management."

For pneumonia, this system reduces diagnosis to looking for only a few physical symptoms. For pneumonia in children, the key is to no-tice when children are breathing fast, or drawing in breath strongly.

The plan in Jumla was to teach volunteers to notice fast or labored breathing, and then watch the child to see if the child took fifty or more breaths per minute. That was the trigger for action.

But counting breath was not a simple matter in Jumla. It required first the ability to count steadily, and second, some way of measuring the time while you count. None of the villagers owned watches or any other easy means of knowing the length of a minute.

The researchers first tried little hourglass-shaped sand timers. But the cheap ones were highly inaccurate and the accurate ones cost more than five dollars each—almost a month's income in Jumla. In the end, they had to invent a simple, cheap timer to give to the villagers.

Their creation was a small electronic beeper that cost three dollars in its early versions. "The Jumla Timer was designed to beep after 30 seconds, since it was found that the difficulty of keeping a child still for a full minute outweighed the slight increase in accuracy which could be gained by a full minute count," the researchers wrote. As it turned out, the timer not only was crucial in determining when to give pills, but when *not* to give pills in the presence of a worried mother.

"In fact," the researchers said, "this strange beeping device soon gained notoriety throughout the district as a supernatural tool capable of judging the cause and severity of a child's cough [and] contributed considerably to a rise in the status of the community health workers using them."

Once the village worker was called to a home, and had tested the child for fast breathing and found it too quick, antibiotic syrup was given for five days. The project weighed the problems of using syrup versus using pills, but came down on the side of the syrup, which was much easier to get children to accept. The mother was given a small bottle of syrup, just enough for the five-days' treatment, and a spoon marked out with the right doses. The mothers were carefully taught how to give the syrup and the importance of using all the medicine in the bottle.

Each of the volunteers in the project was given nine days' training, including role playing and work with actual cases. They were taught not only about treating pneumonia, but how to teach mothers to watch for its signs and the urgency of getting help quickly.

It took more than a year to train the eighty volunteers needed to routinely visit the two hundred villages of Jumla.

The researchers counted the number of deaths and identified their causes throughout the area at the beginning of the study. They found that in the normal way of life, virtually every child got pneumonia every year from birth to age five. Most of the cases, and the worst ones, came during the first year, when children routinely got pneumonia more than once each year.

Sometimes the children were able to fight off the infection, sometimes not. When it came, generally the children lived or died within three and a half days of the appearance of the sickness.

The object of the study was to reduce child deaths in Jumla. They found that by the third year of the project 28 percent fewer deaths were being recorded among them. Most of those saved had been ill with pneumonia. But to the surprise of the researchers, the number of deaths from one or two other causes also dropped somewhat during the period, even though no other services besides the pneumonia project were offered.

The researchers concluded, in a paper published in 1994, that "the study has proven that community health workers are fully capable of carrying out standard pneumonia case management as long as certain programmatic conditions can be met. . . . Substantial reductions in deaths can be achieved even in the complete absence of referral facilities and higher level medical staff."

The study went one step further. After several years of work the researchers added delivery of vitamin A as part of the project. They found that deaths decreased again, beyond the gains from the pneumonia work, now by 5 percent or more.

"Not only were fewer children dying, fewer were getting sick enough with pneumonia to require antibiotic treatment," the researchers said. This meant that ultimately money and time were being *saved* by adding the vitamin supplement to the project.

After the research end of the project ended in the early 1990s, the villages were able to maintain the system and even to add further services. The lower death rates in the area were still being maintained as of the last report in 2002.

One of the interesting lessons learned was that many projects offering education as the first priority have met resistance. The villagers, as the report said, "want action rather than talk. This is a clear example of the necessity to understand the perceived needs of the population to be served."

Because the action and the reduction in deaths came first, the village workers became trusted and were able to bring in less obvious interventions such as vitamin A, and later oral rehydration treatment to prevent deaths from diarrhea. "It made it far easier to introduce oral rehydration," wrote the researchers, "which in many other programs is not readily accepted by families because it is not viewed as medicine and does not cure the most apparent symptoms of diarrhea. Workers have to be believed in order to be effective educators."

It is clear that in difficult places it is not good enough to have a treatment alone. It must be fitted to the environment and introduced in a way the local people can understand and control themselves.

It turns out that the scale of the problem is not the main issue, nor is the large amount of money needed the most important issue. Rather, getting some of the basic medicines and techniques into the hands of local people is vital.

At dusk, Ram and his Western visitors wend their way between huts, stepping over street-running sewage, to talk to a family about their son. Health workers from the neighborhood have heard he has night blindness.

He is about twelve years old and doesn't want to talk about it. But with some nagging from his grandmother, he allows that he has a problem. It's nothing, he says, but as he talks about what the other boys say to him, his eyes tear up. They run around him and call him names. He is worried that he won't be able to do his job, riding the family's water buffalo, guiding him to the field and back.

A crowd is gathering as he talks. On the spot, the boy is given a capsule of vitamin A. The adults surround him and chatter on, while he escapes down the street.

Ram climbs into his truck, and as he drives away, he passes the boy, who is astride his buffalo. The boy's heels knead the beast's ribs to urge him on. Ram smiles and waves. The boy will be better tomorrow, he says.

3

One House at a Time

India Pursues Polio

The single greatest health project in history so far is the current world campaign to eliminate polio. And the great push in this campaign began in October 2004—on one Sunday in India 167 million children were immunized. Within a few days of that, 80 million more children were immunized in Africa. It took 23 million volunteers and troop movement of the scale of multiple-theater operations in World War II.

Yet the whole effort now comes down to a few families in a few neighborhoods in the worst places in the world. That is because of the nature of this particular virus. The trouble is that the virus is easily passed, and it is mostly silent. It infects one hundred to two hundred children for every one that it paralyzes or kills. It cannot be seen easily in those who have it, unlike other diseases such as smallpox. Polio cannot be tracked person to person. So *every* child must be vaccinated. In places where children's immune systems are weak some children need more than one or two rounds of immunization. And of course, even if every child but one were vaccinated on a single day, the one infected child could quickly pass the virus to the new crop of unvaccinated babies being born daily. One case can become ten thousand within months.

Despite the difficulties, the disease is now almost gone. From a time when there were hundreds of thousands of cases of paralysis and death each year, in 2004 there were only 1,266 cases reported worldwide. In 2005, by the end of April, there were only 86.

Now the campaign turns on a few neglected souls and whether they can be reached, physically and mentally.

It is a bright, warm October afternoon in Muzzafarnagar, India. Two young women in brilliantly colored saris pull aside a curtain in an alleyway. It serves as a door to the little yard where a Muslim family lives. There is raw sewage running outside the door. In the darkened interior there is a cow, two pallets, and an array of children.

The young visitors are polio workers. At the beginning of the final worldwide push at the end of 2004, they were going house to house, trying to catch every last child. This little home, and this region of India, are now the crux of the world campaign.

The moment at the door was awkward, confrontational. This family has refused before; they are suspicious. Rumors had run through the neighborhood that the vaccines make children weak, or sterilized them. Two years earlier, when polio workers entered neighborhoods in this area of India, they had been shot at, beaten, and stoned. Now,

Muslim clerics had calmed the disturbances and many had preached in favor of vaccination and publicly prayed for the elimination of polio.

Still, when health workers with nice clothes, sometimes from rich nations, show up, local people may react with something that seems like a mix of anger and self-assertion.

On this October day the leader of the polio workers called out as she pulled the curtain aside, "Hello, can we come in?"

The father and mother of the family emerged from a back room. The woman, holding a baby, said she doesn't want to give the polio medicine to her child. "Please leave."

The head of this family, Ali, complained that health workers never showed up in their neighborhood, no matter how serious the problem. Even when the family travels to the government clinic, they get only bad attitudes and abuse. He wanted to know, what makes you come around chasing after us?

Today, he is clearly irritated that the polio team is back again, this time with supervisors in tow. He is a thirty-four-year-old laborer, and is wearing a dirty, collarless shirt and baggy cotton trousers. He sat down, barefoot, on a small rope pallet.

Hospitality, a universal value here, overcame initial complaints, and soon the young polio volunteers were perched on stools, trying to explain themselves. "Please listen to us. . . . Do you know that by this medicine the child is saved from this handicap?"

"Are you God?" asks Ali.

"No, I don't mean that . . ."

"Answer me! Are you God? We only trust Him."

The young polio worker in blue says, "I come from UNICEF, and I'm from the village, and you know us pretty well."

"That's right. . . . You have only polio in your mind and nothing else," says Ali.

"What do you mean by that?"

"I mean, if any of us here get fever, or other illness, do you give any medicine for that? When we go to hospital, no one gives us medicine." He had explained before about an incident in which he went to the clinic, tried to get treatment, but was shouted at and turned away.

The polio worker presses ahead. "The diseases that you mention . . . [For those] there is medicine we can give after a child is fallen ill. But polio is a disease that cannot be cured once it happens."

"Well, by the grace of God, our child is in good health . . . Allah keeps my child safe. Who are *you* to keep him safe?"

"But," says the young woman, "Allah has given us a brain to think, right? To give medicine is an obligatory act in Islam. Our prophet, peace be upon him, has said this. And now this [medicine] is also Allah's blessing. He gave humans the knowledge to invent a medicine like this."

Ali continues to argue, saying he has lost trust because the government and the doctors do nothing for them.

"I am a Muslim," says the woman in blue. "Would I lie to you? You think I won't come back later?"

Letters they carry from local Islamic authorities soften Ali's position. Finally, he says that because the workers have made the effort to come to his house, and because they ask, he will agree. Soon his small son is trotted out, and the woman in blue tips up his face with her hands, tells him to open his mouth, and two drops of oral vaccine are squeezed in.

The polio crew ducks out through the doorway, and down the path to another dun-colored home, another potential argument.

Difficult as it is to eradicate a single disease from the planet, there is a powerful attraction to try it. The leverage is truly great:

Smallpox was a disease that in medical texts counted as possibly the all-time greatest killer of humanity, and its eradication has been marked as possibly the most cost-beneficial intervention of all time. Hundreds of millions died of it over the three thousand years it ran in waves through society. The campaign to eradicate it began in 1967 and took about twelve years and the aid of about 150 million workers, most of them part-time volunteers. The staff that ran the huge effort comprised 6 medical and logistical officers and 4 secretaries. The total cost of the effort in dollars over twelve years was $300 million.

The nations of the world save about $1.5 billion each year now, as they do not have to diagnose or treat the disease, and do not lose the services of those who are sick or killed by it. The United States alone recovers its part of the cost over and over again, about once every twenty-six days.

There is no stock market or any other kind of investment that can produce such returns for the dollar, never mind the pride of achievement around the world that has come with the work. Smallpox is now the touchstone of thinking in public medicine. How much else can be done for so little? While the approach used to eradicate smallpox may never be duplicated in detail, some principles that made it work have become central to other successful projects since then.

Besides all of that, there is a deep logic here that is appealing. These campaigns use immunization as their chief method. It uses the body's own powers, one by one, person by person, to defeat the disease en masse. It is the ultimate way of helping people help themselves. It cannot be accomplished without the active participation of citizens broadly, and what it offers them is only health—pure opportunity. It is not in itself wealth, or success, but a chance to get up in the morning to go to work, to build, to carry on. It is the purest of devices. And for those who promote this kind of work, it is the simplest bet: that people, given half a chance, will be active, clever, and productive.

This hopeful thinking extends to other immunization campaigns, even if they cannot eradicate their target disease. Many diseases, through routine vaccination of children, can confine illness to small numbers and limited damage.

The first known case of polio was one seen in the withered leg of a scribe, painted on an Egyptian stela about thirty-five hundred years ago. Outbreaks of the disease have been recorded sporadically since then. By 1950, survey work showed there were 210 nations that were routinely swept with epidemics. On average, a thousand children each day were paralyzed and hundreds killed.

Though the virus was everywhere, it tended to come on in bursts, especially in the summertime—such as the outbreak in New York City in 1952, when 57,268 cases were reported, triggering a wave of fear and rounds of ineffective quarantines. Children were prevented from going to public swimming pools and from drinking at public fountains. It was known that the virus is carried by contaminated water, among other things.

But really, it is in that common category of illnesses that move by what doctors delicately call the "fecal-oral" route. That is, those infected excrete the virus in their stool. It can travel through the sewage, and if the water is not treated before reaching a river, lake, or well, the virus will be passed on with the dirty water. But there are other ways the virus can move. If a baby has been infected, and his mother changes his diaper but does not do a good job of washing her hands, the virus can be carried to the next child or into the kitchen. Children in developing countries often defecate in fields or at the roadside, where other feet or hands may wander. Other diseases passed by this route are cholera and the *E. coli* of Jack-in-the-Box fame. The *E. coli* came from cow feces that was accidentally smeared onto other body parts during slaughtering. In another case, cow dung in an apple orchard got onto the skins of fallen apples, and thence into apple juice, triggering a fatal outbreak. It is a natural and easy route for pathogens that need to enter the human body.

And polio does need to enter the human body, because humans are its only host. Once the virus manages to get itself ingested, it makes its way via the digestive system to the cells of the central nervous system, where it multiplies. There, its favored targets are the nerve cells that control muscles. The virus enters the nerve cells, and while multiplying, kills them, thus rendering the muscles without living nerves to control them. The muscles go limp, atrophy, and the limbs become useless appendages. The attack on the nerves happens within a couple of days of infection, beginning with a soreness, fever, and weakness in the limbs. In the worst cases the virus attacks the nerves controlling the muscles for breathing, and death follows quickly. More often, the virus kills the nerves that control the legs. In places where the citizenry have some wealth, this paralysis need not be catastrophic, as the case of Franklin Roosevelt shows. For those without extra resources, however, it means one member of the family who would have been a working, contributing member has suddenly become far less productive, and even a substantial burden on those who must care for him. In human terms, the child—for most polio comes between birth and five years of age—is marked as a figure of debility and ostracism for life.

The first attempt to make vaccines succeeded partially in the 1930s and 1940s, but the first vaccine to be reliable enough to offer to parents was delivered to the United States in a day of widespread celebration in 1955. Then, nation by nation, children were immunized and the disease receded. First, North America became free of it. Many places, however, hadn't the wherewithal to produce a successful national immunization campaign; the disease was cleared only to return again and again to many nations. Canada, the Netherlands, Albania—all countries that had cleared the virus had outbreaks later when the virus came back from still-infected nations. Europe could not shake it until after 2000. And worse, because many countries felt themselves safe, immunizations of young children fell.

By the 1980s it had become clear that nations in Asia and Africa would not be able to eliminate polio on their own, even with one national campaign after another. And that meant a great polio reservoir existed, ready to swarm back across oceans and borders when medical systems became lax and immunization dropped. The world campaign began with the charitable effort of a private group, Rotary International. It succeeded well in the beginning, and then they lobbied the World Health Organization, and finally the official international eradication campaign began in 1988, when there were 350,000 cases in more than one hundred countries.

Now the polio drive is near its end, but the whole effort nearly went off the rails twice: once in India, and once in Nigeria.

By 2001, there had been years of success in India, and only 268 cases. But in 2002, suddenly there were new rumors about America spreading disease against Muslims, and the refusals flared up there. While there were only 92 new cases in the rest of the world, in northern India more than 1,300 new cases were registered in less than a year.

The change was a shock both to Indian health officials and polio campaign leaders at the World Health Organization in Geneva. This sudden upsurge could break the back of the entire global campaign. The message was clear: Something bad is happening on the ground in India, and if you want to beat polio, you must do it here.

The lessons of what happened next are not only about polio but reinforce what we know about what is needed to spur development, to intervene successfully in poor nations.

By the usual human survey methods, the people who are the worst off in society can be difficult to find. Simpler is to follow the polio virus, which can readily find and attack the poorest and most neglected everywhere.

"These are among the most marginalized and most underserved

and underprivileged groups of society," says Sudeep Gadok Singh, one of UNICEF's polio workers. In India, that means not only Muslims, but also low-caste Hindus, the untouchables. (The caste system in northern India is still very much alive and working, and certain professions such as butchers and barbers and laborers are by definition low status.) "They had little or no access to any basic amenities of health, sanitation, and so on. So they had a certain level of mistrust of the local administration. These people were living in ghettoized conditions," he says.

He adds that their isolation had also produced a certain pride and self-sufficiency. "They are self-reliant in their poverty," he says. They were pushed to the point where, on the rare occasions when help was offered, they were ready to refuse.

The concrete form in which poverty produces disease is literally that—concrete. The waste drains out of small pipes directly into the gutters on either side of each alleyway. This is raw sewage, contaminated with all the products of the human gut, most especially the germs of anyone in the neighborhood who is sick. The poor communities are, in the polite term, "underserved." That is, the state health system tends to ignore them almost completely. There are no sewers and no sources of clean water. There are medical clinics, but the people avoid them because of the long waits and abusive treatment. There is a joke told when asked about the local health clinic. In India, people are familiar with rabies caught from dog bites, and the insanity that comes with the disease. When asked why they don't go to the local clinic, they reply with their version of, You think I'm crazy?: "What? Have I been bitten by a dog, that I should go to the clinic?"

So when polio volunteers show up at their door talking about health, the locals are surprised and suspicious.

In the poor nations, Western workers don't often show up at the doors of the poor and minorities. The last time many remember—and have created stories about—was the family planning workers of the 1970s. There was always a suspicion that "birth control" programs were mainly aimed at curtailing the rising population of minorities. Sterilization was a common birth control method, and it added to the fear of a conspiracy, already well ingrained by the neglect they were suffering from their own government.

The minorities became suspicious again when the polio teams, usually including a number of Americans, began intensive work, moving from village to village.

"Look at it this way," says David Heymann, chief of the world polio eradication program for the World Health Organization. As a young man, he had been one of those who labored in India to eradicate smallpox, and was now back to finish off polio. "When you have a vaccine and deliver it to a household in a village where children are dying from malaria or some other disease and can't get medicines, there's going to be suspicion." Heymann reflects on the attitudes he has encountered. "Why is the government bringing me this when everything else, they don't have? And why do they keep bringing this every month? Why is it so important to them? Why are Europeans coming with them? This raises suspicions in their minds, and would in anyone's mind."

Jay Wenger, chief of the National Polio Surveillance Project of India and WHO, housed in a warren of offices under the stands at

Nehru Stadium in Delhi, names a couple of points from their failure analysis. The districts in western Uttar Pradesh province, being poor and Muslim, are not welcome postings for the mostly Hindu state medical officials. A survey of the top health jobs in each district found that those of district medical officer and chief nurse were routinely left vacant in more than half of the poor areas. These were the medical people who were to work with UNICEF and WHO in organizing polio teams. They were supposed to be the Indian government's on-the-ground leaders, but they simply did not exist.

They also found that in the poor areas the vaccinator teams were too often two men, both Hindus, whose job it was to walk into Muslim neighborhoods and knock on doors. In Muslim households, the women by tradition do not open the door to strange men while the heads of the household are away. That meant the polio workers had no access to whole neighborhoods. Even when the local inhabitants were not reluctant, some of the polio volunteers were. Some did not want to go into the alleys of the poor districts. The teams were supposed to have at least one member from the community that was being visited, but in many cases this had not happened. That meant that the fear and suspicion between peoples was intruding during the polio canvassing, and progress had stopped.

After their research on the failures of 2002, polio workers in India had systematically met with and questioned local people in poor communities about their feelings, not just on polio, but on other health matters. They ended up listening to long litanies of people's general dissatisfaction. And to conclude, the villagers wondered aloud why only the polio vaccine was being offered. What about help with the main killers in their neighborhoods—diarrhea, tuberculosis, pneumonia?

Two young men, Sudeep Gadok Singh and Naysan Sahba, are traveling together today, in fall 2004, in Aligarh, a town about a hundred kilometers south of Delhi's great urban sprawl. Sahba and Singh are both in jeans; one is wearing a turban, the other a UNICEF baseball cap.

The two men are here, up early each day and driving from spot to spot, because this is the day, the great push to immunize the Indian population—not gradually, but all at once, on a single day. And they are here because this place is the worst case. They need to work here hardest.

Decades ago when smallpox was finally scrubbed from the human population, there were two or three spots where the last cases were found. This was one of them. Polio has three viral types. Type 2 has been eliminated as a human disease. The last case was also found here in Aligarh. When, two years ago, there was a sudden outbreak of new polio cases around the world, this single province in India had twice as many cases as all the rest of the world combined. As disease sinks go, this is a tough place.

A brief glimpse of the town would suggest it had been bombed heavily. Brick walls are half standing. Pools of water and muck are everywhere. There is trash in the road and in drifts up against the walls.

But actually, it's more like a slow-motion construction site. The people inhabiting the ruins of brick and concrete, while they cannot afford to buy many bricks, scavenge them and pile them up gradually to make walls for their houses. The walls are not partly down, they are partly up.

The low level of life around them is not only usual for the two men, they take it as a sort of challenge: We know people should not live like this; let's do something. The pair are of a type that can be found around the world in tough places. They are smart and educated and of all nationalities. They constitute the spiritual descendants of the Peace Corps of earlier days, or perhaps the nineteenth-century missionaries and sanitary reformers. The have a sense of humor, and optimism, and easiness with many different sorts of people. They may work for charitable groups or health groups or antipoverty projects.

Sahba and Singh are with UNICEF, the United Nations Children's Fund, and its campaign to eradicate the polio virus.

Naysan Sahba was born in Iran, raised in India, and carries a Canadian accent and passport. His father was an architect who designed the two greatest temples of the Baha'i faith in Israel and Canada. Naysan, a Baha'i, found his strongest enthusiasm early in life was for drama. In college he wrote papers describing how to use drama to link different cultures to the key goals of development and progress. He worked in Latin America, and then in Israel, then organizing ceremonies and events for the World Health Organization. Two years ago he was posted to India in the state of Uttar Pradesh, as a lieutenant in the war on polio. By 2004, he is married, with a six-month-old, and his wife is an interior designer who is able to make a living in the ancient Indian capital of Lucknow in Uttar Pradesh, where they now live.

Sudeep Gadok Singh is, he says with a grin, "just a Sikh guy." His family is from the Punjab region that is now split between India and Pakistan. He wears the wrapped Sikh turban, in dark blue, above a black beard. He is an MD, but routinely wears jeans and a T-shirt. Among his favorite fashion non sequiturs is to wear a "capitalist" T-shirt (Lee Jeans in big letters) above a socialist belt buckle (a brass hammer and sickle). He is twenty-eight years old, full of energy and flair. He says his credentials for his job as a "commander" of polio volunteers comes in his genes—his father is a colonel in the army and his mother is a doctor. As he strolls down an alleyway, he will spot a child, reach over to brush his hair and chat with him. Then the query: "Did you get your polio drops?"

The effort to take on the final few houses with polio produced a different strategy than the eradication campaign had started with, and the difference was significant. Originally, it was planned that polio booths would be set up in villages and local people would be invited out to get their children immunized. This approach had already worked in most of the world, including most of the states of India.

But in the most difficult places, house to house, person to person outreach, with carefully thought-out messages (and messengers) would be necessary.

This is important because it hits on a point debated for many years by those who work in developing countries. Two strategies have been used over the years—the "vertical" in which money and experts from the outside come into a country, carry out a program with local help, and then leave. The other approach is called "horizontal," in which the object is to build up the local clinics and skills of local workers, and put them in place to deal with a variety of health and wealth problems.

They are intended to be sustainable and to become functioning local institutions.

There are reasons why both approaches exist, and both have worked in various ways. Each has its drawbacks as well.

But what the polio campaign showed was a vertical program turning into a horizontal program on the ground in a few places when difficult local issues arose.

This time in India the polio campaign workers made sure the house-to-house teams had both women and Muslims, and that in the high-risk areas one member of the two-member teams lived in the neighborhood they were canvassing, said Naysan Sahba. They also went on to recruit "influencers" from each neighborhood—the leader of a madrassa, a successful businessman, the top local politician. They would be recruited to attend local meetings, to give talks at rallies, to inaugurate polio booths on immunization day. There were, of course, the top soccer star in India and the most popular Bollywood actors as well. Their endorsements—surrounded by folk music and a patter—were used in pressing points during door-to-door work. They were also broadcast from the minarets in mosques, after prayer call, and from loudspeakers on the backs of rickshaws moving through the markets.

The polio workers convinced the government to bring in medical officers from around India to help fill the jobs, and more, in high-risk districts name not just one, but three, four, or five medical officers to press the work.

The five hundred are not paid regular wages but less than half a month's pay for each month's work, so they are, more or less, volunteers. They have some other reason to be there than making money. The workers go out in pairs and are assigned neighborhoods, and given detailed plans about how to work them.

The teams go out to each house more than once, taking with them information about other medical issues besides polio. They talk pregnancy and child rearing. They sometimes help make appointments and offer transport to local clinics. They carry charts with routine immunization facts. They have flip charts with pictures to explain immunization and why each child must get a dose each round. The polio volunteers have been trained to give some other health advice, chiefly on pregnancy and childhood problems. They can also bring children and families to the clinic and make sure they are seen.

And, in the days before Immunization Day, each community is treated to a health camp. At the health camp, on one day from morning until evening a doctor, a nurse, a pharmacist, and others come to the neighborhood with a full box of advice and medicines—from antibiotics to salves to contraceptives, which are provided free. "We want them to know we care about things besides polio. We want to connect with them," says Naysan as he stands by a great pink and yellow curtain at one health camp setup. Four tables are placed beneath a water tower, given the colored cloths as a backdrop, and the clinic is underway.

"We explain it by talking about the kid," Singh says. "We say the kid is like a house. The virus and the vaccine are enemies and can't live in the house together. If the virus lives in a kid, and the vaccine enters, the virus is thrown out. Once it is thrown out of that house, it can't survive for long. So we are trying to throw out the virus from all its houses at once, so that it falls into the street and perishes quickly and can't get back in." In Aligarh district alone there were health camps offered in 113 neighborhoods.

Other special efforts were added. In the ten days before Immunization Day there were also cleanup days. Singh's districts, including Aligarh and Moradabad, had been the worst of the worst. Now he was leading a small army of five hundred in those areas.

On the big day itself, polio workers are up and out between 4:00 and 5:00 A.M. The first stop that Sunday is the district hospital, Malkhan Singh Hospital.

The vaccine vials for the whole district are to be delivered by 5:00 A.M. The small plastic bottles of vaccine, about two inches high, hold about forty drops, or twenty doses, of polio vaccine each. There are small gray picnic coolers, hundreds of them, waiting and filled with dry ice. About fifteen of the plastic vials will be packed in each. Then each cooler will be delivered to a designated spot in town and farmland by four-wheel-drive Mahindra "jeeps." (The tarred roads are bad enough, but the smaller roads leading to villages, especially after a rain, can be nearly impassable even with four-wheel drive.) Volunteers wait for the drop-offs, and will take the gray coolers to their "polio booths."

During the week before the big day, there was a media blitz. Banners were strung across streets and draped from walls. Posters were pasted by the dozen on poles and buildings. Naysan Sahba, who was leading the information campaign, pointed out that while towns like

Aligarh are poor in many other ways, they are not lacking in pitches. If you close your eyes, turn around, and spit randomly, he said, you'll hit an ad. They cover all surfaces and remain even as reminders in the froth along the sewage troughs. So, an intense effort is needed.

In the few days before booth day, troops of folk performers—159 of them giving 2,000 performances—traveled the towns and villages putting up polio banners and staging magic shows, folk music concerts, puppet shows, and other assorted theatrical events. There were rallies at schools, marches down the alleyways with banners in the afternoons, and nighttime parades with torches and the shouting of the polio slogans.

At the same time as the blitz, volunteers in the worst areas moved house-to-house in searches for all the unvaccinated children. They've mapped every house, counted and recorded every child.

"It's not an option," said Sahba, "we have to reach every child." For every case of paralysis, there are a hundred or more "silent" polio infections. These cases may produce only mild fever and weakness, but they are able to spread the virus just as effectively as those totally paralyzed by it. But in this part of India no one has ever really tried to reach every family, every child to deliver some service, any service. This is the home of the masses, and in particular the mass of ignored minorities.

Just as the newly reorganized campaigns started in India outbreaks of polio exploded thousands of miles away—in Nigeria. The rumors of sterilization and other resistance that had sprouted in India had now reached Muslim neighborhoods in Africa, and the poor, marginalized

Muslims there began to refuse to have their children vaccinated. The vaccine, it was said, was yet another plot by the government and the West, leading to sterilization or AIDS.

In Nigeria, as in India, the countryside is split along religious and cultural lines. Muslims and Christians are at odds. The national leadership governs from the south and central parts of the country and comprises 40 percent of the population, while Muslims live in the north and are about 50 percent of the national population. For a long time, however, the Muslims have complained of abuse from the government, and there has been a series of violent clashes between Christians and Muslims.

Sometime during 2002 rumors began to spread, possibly from India via the Internet. Then, suddenly, the rumors gained verification from government officials in Nigeria. The Muslim leadership in Kano state in the north announced that they believed the polio vaccine was contaminated with birth control drugs. A state laboratory in Kano— the leading Muslim region in Nigeria—had done a little analysis of the vaccine, and apparently found some contamination. The chemical they found, though in tiny amounts, was said to be related to estrogen, the female hormone used in contraceptives. The finding was not confirmed by other labs, and vaccine officials and manufacturers quickly said that whatever was found was likely to be just a trace contamination with no biological effect.

But a political effect, it did have. A Muslim doctor, Ibrahim Datti Ahmed, secretary general of the Supreme Council for Shariah in Nigeria, told reporters, "It's not a contamination, it's adulteration. It's an attempt to control the population of the Third World."

Three Nigerian states (Kano, Zamfara, and Kaduna) shut down the polio vaccination program in the summer of 2003. Sule Ya'u Sule, a spokesman for Kano state, said that Kano scientists "made the discovery of the contaminants," and that Kano would not participate in any more vaccinations "unless we are convinced by our committee [of health experts] that the oral polio vaccines are safe. The exercise remains suspended in Kano."

The WHO and the Nigerian government sponsored tests of the vaccine that showed it contained no contraceptives or contaminants related to them. But those tests, done in labs in Geneva, Lagos, and elsewhere in Nigeria, were rejected by the Muslim officials in the north. They said they were suspicious and wanted their own tests by a laboratory of their choosing in a Muslim country. While the debate went on, polio was moving.

In 2001, the disease had been suppressed by vaccination, from thousands of cases annually in the 1980s to only 56 cases throughout Nigeria in 2001. The year the rumors began, 2002, the cases shot up to 202, and after the Muslim authorities halted vaccination the number of those paralyzed went up to 355. Nigeria became the only polio-endemic nation that stopped vaccinating. Worse, the disease, which had largely been contained in the north, broke out again and was reinfecting not only other parts of Nigeria that had rid themselves of polio, but other African nations as well. By 2004, twelve African nations that had eliminated the virus were again infected with cases that were genetically determined to have originated in Nigeria.

Reporters visiting Nigeria began to document the cases. John Donnelly of the *Boston Globe* went to Kano and villages in the north.

He wrote that the leaders in the region had told their followers not to accept the vaccine, and that its use was an American plot against Islam.

> *Some leaders admitted in interviews late last year [2003] that they never believed such a thing. But they remained silent, they said, in order to stop anything associated with the United States— the U.S.-led wars in Iraq and Afghanistan, several said, had led them to believe that America wants to control the Islamic world, and the polio vaccination effort gave them an opportunity to resist a U.S.-funded initiative.... "People believe that America hates Muslims, and so whatever comes from the United States, no matter how good it is, people will reject it," said Sheik Muhammed Nasir Muhammed, the chief imam at the second largest mosque in Kano.*

There are perhaps three thousand souls in the village of Batakaye, where, Donnelly wrote, four fresh cases of polio had appeared after the vaccinations were stopped. When Donnelly arrived the Muslim families said they would welcome the vaccine. One community leader said that while opinions about Americans are now divided, the opinions about the vaccine were not, because the four cases in the small village after years without a case were proof enough.

Naturally, when it was time for Kamzullahi Sha'aibu, one year old, to get his vaccination, the family decided it was best not to bring him to the clinic after the edict of their imam. Later, after the drops in the mouth were refused, one afternoon Sha'aibu became sick. Not long afterward he was overcome by weakness and fever. Within days, his left leg and right arm became paralyzed. Abdul Kareem Sha'aibu, the boy's father, now takes care of him, bringing him to therapy once a week in a village five miles away. "What happened was an act of God," Sha'aibu said. "When they come around with the vaccine again, all our children will take it. They see Kamzullahi, and the other three children. But I haven't given up on my child. I am optimistic he will walk again, God willing."

It was not until June 2004, almost a year after the ban on vaccination, that the governor of Kano relented and permitted vaccination again. By that time it was too late to stop the new outbreak, and the number of cases continued to rise to more than 650 in Nigeria, with a hundred fresh cases in other African nations as well.

The Nigerian Muslim leaders said they were now determined to stop polio again. In a ceremony at a stadium and before a large crowd, Governor Ibrahim Shekarau, the man who had ordered the end of vaccination, now said he was "satisfied with the process of production" of the vaccine. "Our argument has been we wanted scientific proof." Now, he said, he had it, after a laboratory in Indonesia, the fourth round of tests of the vaccine, said it was free of contamination.

By October 2004, the Nigerians and the Indians were both ready to try again.

On October 10 in Aligarh, India, 314 polio booths are set up, each manned by three people. In the rest of Uttar Pradesh province are another 3,400 workers and booths.

The "booths" are nothing more than a table, a few chairs, and an array of red and yellow banners announcing the great polio day. Children under five will be brought to the booth, given two drops of polio vaccine by mouth, and although their names are not taken, a check mark will yield numbers at the end of the day to cross-check against the number of doses given out. After getting the drops, each child's left little finger is marked on the nail and cuticle with an indelible black mark that will last for more than a week.

In some states in India, as well as in other countries, more than 90 percent of the children can be vaccinated just through a well-organized booth day. The mothers and children will come out. But in Aligarh, only about 45 percent of the children can be reached that way. So this time, for two weeks after booth day teams of vaccinators will scour the neighborhoods, door-to-door, trying to find any child without a black pinkie.

As he moves from booth to booth checking how the volunteers are doing, examining their records and testing their training, Sahba muses about the society around him. It is more vibrant in some ways than most any other place on earth, he says. "It is sort of inside-out. In other places all the making and doing and selling go on inside gray buildings behind walls. But here, everything is on the outside, spilling into the streets." The tea shops fry roti bread out front; the men with hammers beat tires in the dust in front of their shops. The merchandise—TVs to goats' heads—sits on the countertops. There must be more small businesses here per square foot than any other place on earth.

In one street, the polio booth was set up outside the front door of the school called "National Public School" in green and red. The area is a slum called Shah Jamal, after a great leader of three or four centuries ago. At this little booth, by 10:30 A.M., 117 children have been immunized. Watching for a moment it is clear that it is not often the mothers who bring the children in; it is the older brothers and sisters carrying their struggling and gangly younger sibs to the table.

At the next stop the polio booth is set up in the doorway of a "quack" shop (the word quack is *not* derogatory here) called the "Saifi Medical Institute of Electropathy for the promotion, development and research of electropathy, S. U. Saifi, principal." By 11:23 in the morning 230 children had been immunized here. Across the street is a playground with puddles and a sewer beside it. "Playground for the virus, more like," says Sahba as he walks by.

There are also three booths in the main railway station in Aligarh. One percent of all children in India this Sunday will be aboard trains, but nonetheless, they cannot be missed. At one booth, 130 have been treated, but out on the train platform itself, though crowds sit on the pavement awaiting trains, only 72 children have been vaccinated.

Singh and Sahba corner the young woman who is supposed to be combing the crowds. They chastise her mildly and then bring her out along the platform, showing her how to greet the families one by one and ask about vaccination. Then, as train 31110 pulls in, Singh hops aboard the train and walks down the aisle, greeting the families. He spots a young girl in red, with white lace. With a smile he pats her head and picks up her pinkie. No mark. He asks the parents, they nod, and quickly a vial is out and two drops are in the girl's mouth as her eyes go wide. Within fifteen or twenty minutes of arrival, the team has logged fifteen more children.

Later, the team is out in the countryside, rural Aligarh. In one area called Jawam, they visit Samera village, a couple of kilometers from anything else in sight besides sugarcane. There at the end of a lane is a walled-in yard with a bright yellow polio banner. They have logged 202 children so far. But here there is some potential trouble. The cold box is open, and the vials are getting warm. The little bottles have a chemical in a mark on the side; as it is exposed to light and warmth, it goes gray. At a certain tone it is no longer to be used. One of the vials here has gone gray and the volunteers had not noticed. They didn't understand about the "cold box" that had to keep the vaccine below 8°C. It is soon discovered that some of the workers were not trained, and the immunization campaign for the whole neighborhood was at risk.

At times during the day, both Singh and Sahba could be seen gesticulating, arguing, even shouting that some of the volunteers were not up to their jobs. But by the end of the day, as the sun was turning a gray haze in the sky to brilliant pink, they were silent riding back into the center of town.

A reporter asks Singh whether they would succeed. Would they clear the virus from this landscape?

He tells a story passed down by health volunteers from the days of smallpox. Some of those early volunteers were energetic and smart, but not too presentable. They had long hair and sloppy clothes. "You couldn't take them to cocktail parties. But they succeeded. When asked how, [the volunteers] were told that the young, hippie-looking doctors were filled with a fierce, unwarranted optimism," Singh says, and laughs. "So now that's me. I am filled with unwarranted optimism. Yes, yes. We will do it."

4

Changing Minds

Botswana Beats Back AIDS

The greatest public health challenge in our time is AIDS, and the place it has wreaked the most havoc is in Africa. Sub-Saharan Africa has about 10 percent of the world's people, but about 60 percent of the people infected with HIV; in more than a dozen countries, it has become common practice to hire two or even three people to fill each job because of the certainty that workers will die within a short time after training. About 26 million people in Southern Africa are infected now, and that means, even with future successes, the epidemic will be a major presence for many years to come. If a new global health campaign is to be waged, the defeat of AIDS in Africa must be a priority. The myths about AIDS in Africa persist—that money to fight AIDS is lost to corruption, that Africans have resisted condoms and behavior change more than others. The truth is progress has been made in several places in Africa, and much more progress is expected as sophisticated HIV treatments become more accessible to Africans. The most remarkable case of progress against HIV in Africa has been in

Botswana, which is now leading what has been called the "decade of treatment" in Africa.

Whoever called Africa the dark continent must have been blind, because there is very little of Africa that could be called dark. Here in the great southern expanses of the continent, day after day, the sky is empty of clouds; intense light fills the whole blue bowl.

The morning is cool and promising; then the day opens itself up and heat and light pour in like a hot liquid. The searing brightness drives cows, goats, people, and cars under trees for shade. But the evening forgives sins and cools again, relenting in a mild night amid the perfume of wood smoke and flowering trees.

Tucked away hundreds of kilometers from the coasts, Botswana is said to be the last remnant of ancient Africa, the last open wilderness on the continent. Despite the depredations of the times, forty-five thousand elephants still roam in herds in this country. The lions, zebras, and giraffes move freely on great expanses of savannah. This place was largely unreached by the colonial thrust 120 years ago from all the coasts inward. Botswana writer Bessie Head said that Botswana has always been a bit apart from the fray. "A bit of ancient Africa was left almost intact to dream along its own way."

When Botswana was declared independent in 1966 its prospects were grim. It was one of the two or three poorest nations in the world, with its citizens earning fewer than two dollars per day, and nothing to give hope for more.

It sits up on high tableland, grass and bush savannah mostly, with a great desert—the Kalahari—in the middle and west of the country. There is too little rain for agriculture in most of the country, just enough to grow grasses for cattle. At the time of independence, the nation, the size of Texas, had a total of four miles of road, essentially no electricity, and no telephones. The airport was a dirt strip with a shack sometimes housing an attendant. From the shack it was a hefty hike to the new capital city, Gaborone.

But from that low state, everything changed. Diamonds were unearthed soon after; the best and purest cache in the world lay beneath the country's red and ochre soil. Many nations have rich resources and squander them; not so in Botswana. The government planned wisely and built a parliamentary democracy strong on merit and clean of corruption. With the diamond money the government built schools, roads, clinics, and wells across the dry nation.

Botswana soon was the star of Africa—with the highest growth rate in the world, 9.2 percent—between 1966 and 1996. Average life spans shot up over a similar period, from 46 to 67.5 years expectancy in 1999. School enrollment went up from about 40 percent of children to 98.4 percent. Literacy went up to over 80 percent, among men and women equally. Ninety-seven percent of the Batswana have safe drinking water within 2.5 kilometers of home. Child immunization for five diseases rose to up over 95 percent.

There were problems amid the prosperity, of course. The wealth was not evenly divided. Wealth is measured in cattle in Botswana, and a little over 2.5 percent of Batswana own 40 percent of the nation's cattle. Two-thirds of the women and one-third of the men have no cattle at all. In a country with no industry and very tough farming, that is serious. Even in the midst of prosperity, unemployment remained high—it's estimated to be 40 percent. Half the people still earn less than a dollar a day, though because land is communally held and essentially free for citizens, most everyone has a place to go to lay her head, even if it's only a hut on parched ground.

At first, it looked like the horseman of pestilence would pass Botswana by. The epidemic of AIDS flared up in the United States, then in the Caribbean, then Europe, and finally it became its most intense across a belt in the middle of Africa, from Kenya to Uganda and down to Zambia. Until about 1993, Botswana was spared.

Then the epidemic struck hard, like a silent storm sweeping down the eastern boundary of the nation, dropping an unwelcome viral rain. By 2000, Botswana found itself with almost 40 percent of its adult population infected with HIV, one of the highest rates of infection ever recorded for any disease. Some towns had even higher rates—up to 52 percent in one town that serves as a way station on the truck route from Zimbabwe.

This small, successful country thus became the worst spot in what is arguably the worst epidemic in human history. The people, led by President Festus Mogae, an Oxford-trained development economist and a former official of the World Bank, began to worry about the future of the nation. As Mogae himself said, this is the worst thing that had ever happened there, bar none.

Just as matters got to their worst, a plan emerged.

The bold project in Botswana started with an idea inside the executive offices at Merck & Co. in Whitehouse Station, New Jersey, in talks with experts at the Harvard AIDS Institute and Harvard University.

The plan was to tackle an entire nation at once. Too many AIDS projects were short or limited to one aspect of the problem, such as counseling for those infected, or providing condoms, or writing educational materials. Why not take one nation and try to provide a complete set of services, from education in schools to prevention messages in the media, to condom distribution, to testing for HIV, to counseling, to full AIDS treatment in hospitals and clinics? It would be most unusual particularly because it would offer sophisticated triple-drug AIDS treatments to all the people of the nation, free of charge, permanently. Could such a comprehensive effort turn back the epidemic? That was the bet.

Merck was at the top of the pharmaceutical industry, hugely profitable. But there was trouble ahead; the entire pharmaceutical industry was beginning a terrible slide in the eyes of the public.

The drugs beginning to come on the market in 1996 were the greatest breakthrough in AIDS treatment since the beginning of the epidemic. They were a new category of drugs called "protease inhibitors." These, combined with earlier drugs, made a potent antiviral "cocktail."

The excitement over the drugs was uncontainable. Even before they were released patients were clamoring for them. People who had three hundred thousand to a million virus particles per deciliter of their blood found that the drugs knocked those counts to zero. Some small numbers of viruses undoubtedly remained, but they could not be detected.

The physical consequences of it was dramatic. Lazarus stories began to be reported of patients who were within days or hours of death when they got the drugs. Two weeks later they were up and about, gaining weight and getting ready to go back to work. Over time, the miracle was confirmed. As many as 90 percent of those infected were able to knock out the virus and restart their lives; it is now estimated that the drugs can add ten, and possibly many more, healthy years onto the life of an infected person.

There were fifty-one thousand deaths from AIDS in the United States in 1995. After the drugs appeared in the United States the death rate dropped immediately and soon was down to fifteen thousand per year, and is still dropping in 2005. Doctors are cautious about pronouncements like this, but they began to say that near normal life spans might be ahead for many of those infected with HIV.

The industry had avoided getting into the business of researching and producing AIDS drugs. But when they did, the companies made a strategic blunder. They decided to set prices for AIDS drugs at extremely high levels, enough to produce gasps even in the business press.

These drugs were true lifesavers. But the companies set their prices between ten and fifteen thousand dollars per person for a year's supply. That did not take into account the other thousands of dollars needed for medicines and doctors by people infected with HIV, and it was a price that would have to be paid every year into the future.

Worse, when the companies were asked to send the drugs to Africa and Asia for cheaper prices, they flatly refused. They feared that if there were two prices their arguments that high prices were justified would be undermined. Soon, generic manufacturers were defying Western patents and making the drug cocktails for less than $150 for a year's supply *and still making a profit*. Thus it was clear just how inflated the Western drug company prices were.

The companies made further blunders, arguing that a good price wouldn't matter in Africa because those countries didn't have the infrastructure—doctors and clinics and refrigerators—to handle proper distribution of the drugs anyway, so high prices weren't important.

Famously, Andrew Natsios, the head of the U.S. Agency for International Development, testified in Congress that Africans shouldn't get the drugs.

> *If we had [the drugs] today, we could not distribute them. We could not administer the program because we do not have the doctors, we do not have the roads, we do not have the cold chain. . . . If you have traveled to rural Africa you know this, this is not a criticism, just a different world. People do not know what watches and clocks are. They do not use western means for telling the time. They use the sun. These drugs have to be administered during a certain sequence of time during the day and when you say take it at 10:00, people will say, what do you mean by 10:00?*

The argument was made that if the drugs were not taken properly, and doses were missed, then the virus could quickly become resistant. That could render them useless for all.

The reaction to all this was outrage. A Harris poll showed that the drug companies were popular and respected up until 1997, when their rating by the public was 79 percent favorable. By 2000, it had dropped to 59 percent, and did not stop there. By 2004 it had sunk to 44 percent favorable and 48 percent unfavorable. People were now saying the companies were greedy and drug prices were too high. No industry in the poll's history had ever fallen so far and so fast in the public esteem.

Roy Vagelos, by then former chairman of Merck, began to condemn the companies outright. "This industry delivered miracles, and now they're throwing it all away," he said. "They just don't get it." As if to reinforce Vagelos's comments, Pat Kelly, president of Pfizer's American drug division, said when told the drug companies were now esteemed as low as cigarette companies, "We find it incredible that we could be equated to an industry that kills people as opposed to cures them."

Poorer nations said that they could not afford the drugs, but they had real AIDS emergencies and they had no choice but to seize the formulas for the drugs and make cheap copies themselves to give to their people. Brazil and India started making and using emergency "generic" AIDS drugs. In South Africa the law allowed the government to force pharmaceutical companies to grant licenses for making the drugs during an emergency. The drug companies took the South African government to court to maintain control over the drugs and their prices; and the companies lost.

Merck officials were feeling the pinch of the criticism. This was particularly difficult for Merck, which had a reputation for charitable instincts, and its executives routinely quoted their founder's remarks about how health was first and profits second.

The company had just succeeded in a philanthropic venture that was the most remarkable in the history of the pharmaceutical industry. The company has a drug that is a very powerful antiparasite medicine; it was the top seller among veterinary drugs. Scientists inside the company knew that it would also be useful against parasites in humans, but unfortunately the humans infected with parasites were not in major markets. The patients who needed the drug couldn't pay the price, so Merck at first did not make a human version of it.

In the end, Merck decided to make the drug and donate it to the people who needed it. Further, they offered to create a delivery system. By the late 1990s 25 million people per year were getting the drug. Some areas, where half the people had in the past been infected with river blindness now saw essentially no cases. (River blindness is a parasitic disease passed by the bites of black flies: the flies thrive near rivers which are also the most fertile farmland, but which must be abandoned for higher ground when too many people go blind from the bites.) The gains turned out to be more than health. Farm output jumped up, as people were able to work more and in areas previously off-limits because of infestations of worm-carrying black flies.

Another Merck project done in combination with the Harvard AIDS Institute was the "enhancing care initiative," a project to understand how best to deliver AIDS care in developing countries. It soon became clear that piecemeal projects by universities, NGOs, and governments, with poor communication among the groups, would be ineffective in addressing the epidemic.

Gradually, Merck executives and Harvard public health doctors were learning that even if the price problem could be resolved, the harder issue would be finding ways of delivering the drugs. "Improving infrastructure was key to making a difference in HIV," said Guy Macdonald, then Merck vice president. "Just donating drugs is not enough." He said it was frustrating that the public debate was about unconscionable prices, when he knew that even if the prices drop to zero, the drugs still would not get to the people who need them.

Macdonald and other executives had become so isolated from mainstream opinion that they had lost sight of the main point—whether AIDS was a tough problem in other ways wasn't the issue. Setting high prices was an act that on its own was unconscionable.

In the middle of the public relations crisis over AIDS drug prices, in August 1999, Macdonald went to a Merck management committee saying that Merck should go beyond the previous "enhancing care" project and do something bolder on AIDS. The Gates Foundation surprised Merck by offering to put in $50 million if Merck would match it. So, the scale of the project was set at $100 million, to be spent over five years in some nation that needed an anti-HIV program.

The five countries that on paper appeared to be the best candidates were those in Africa hard-hit by HIV—Uganda, Malawi, Senegal, Rwanda, and Botswana. The country chosen had to have both an HIV problem and, far more important, a government willing to tackle it. That left out many countries immediately, most especially South Africa, where the government refused to build an AIDS treatment program and rejected Western drugs.

Botswana was the smallest and likely the most manageable spot for a project. What decided the matter finally was President Festus Mogae, who told Merck and Gates at their first meeting that the project should have started yesterday; a sense of urgency was needed.

Then CEO Ray Gilmartin and Vice President Guy Mcdonald made the announcement on July 10, 2000.

What began in Botswana in 2000 soon grew into the most important experiment on AIDS ever done. No one had tackled an entire nation before with a comprehensive program including the most sophisticated AIDS drugs, especially not in Africa. It became the largest and longest running public health project on the African continent.

It was also in a new and growing category of aid, called "public-private partnerships," in which international private groups become partners with governments to carry out large projects.

The plan raised startlingly clear questions: It was said the price of the drugs was killing tens of thousands—what if the drugs were free? It was said that even if the drugs were shipped to developing nations, they could not get them to patients because governments were ineffective. It was said that even if the drugs were offered on all street corners, people wouldn't take them because they did not even want to know if they were infected, and besides they didn't believe in Western treatments. This bold project would answer those questions and more.

Why Botswana? It seems strange that such a small, peaceful country should be the center of a firestorm, the nation to reach the highest level of infection anywhere on earth. People puzzled over it for a few years, from a dozen different perspectives.

It was an unusual conjunction of three dark stars over the time and the place—unusual happenings in love, in the virus itself, and in the movement of the people along the roads that made the difference.

First, one of the worst pieces of biological news in recent decades has been the finding that HIV changes routinely. Gene trading with other bugs, it has developed a new, more troublesome strain in southern Africa. The viral type that began the HIV epidemic in America, Africa, and Europe in the early 1980s was one that came to be called HIV-1b. The kinds most common in Central and East Africa have been HIV-1a and HIV-1d. Only a decade later did a new one, HIV-1c, spread in southern Africa. This one spreads and multiplies faster than any previous type. Upon genetic examination, it has been found to have at least two features that make it more dangerous than its predecessors. First, it has an ability to latch onto the surface of vaginal and penile skin cells more readily than other strains. Second, it multiplies more readily than other strains. More particles more able to attach to skin cells may make the C strain more adept at spreading.

At the peak of the epidemic in Uganda, 15 to 20 percent of pregnant women, who are the sentinel group, were infected at the peak of the epidemic in Uganda with A and D types. But in the countries infected with the C type the rates are double and triple that.

A second feature of the epidemic alighting in southern Africa is that the people in Botswana and neighboring areas are extremely mobile for people of a traditional culture. They move constantly, from farm to cattle post to city and back again, thus assuring that couples are constantly apart and vulnerable to second loves.

This mobility is at least partly a legacy of colonialism. When the British were making colonies all around Botswana, they needed labor. The solution was to impose a "hut tax" on the Tswana tribes, payable only in British money. People who would normally pay in cattle or goats were thus forced to get "paying" work. That paying work, of course, was not in their local villages. It was in the mines of South

Africa, or on distant estates of white settlers. So the Batswana got used to husbands on the move and family members in general traveling to get work.

The impact of this high mobility is that there is no settled family life. Typically, mothers and fathers do not raise their children themselves; grandmothers and aunts raise the children. Young couples are often away from each other, and during these times they develop other relationships.

This leads to the most important reason why AIDS in southern Africa runs at a higher rate: It is fractured relationships. Not sex, but relationships.

Despite the mythology to the contrary, Africans are not more promiscuous than other people. As researchers have discovered in recent years, the term "promiscuity" has little meaning in the real world, as patterns of behavior are mixed everywhere.

Relationships and sex are different. To start with the sexual habits of two rather different groups—Americans and Batswana—it is clear that the Batswana are in general *not* more promiscuous. Studies show that the peoples with the greatest number of sexual partners are the Americans, French, and Germans, while Asians and Africans lag in both the number of partners and the frequency of sex. The Americans have more sexual partners than the Africans do, and their sexual adventures are more abrupt—more one-night stands and sudden runs of activity. The number of sex partners is not the essential problem in southern Africa. It is something more fundamental.

In traditional Africa the basic standard is, in fact, the standard of the Old Testament. Faithfulness is valued, but male authority is paramount. A man who is prosperous enough traditionally may have a mistress or a second wife, as in the Bible.

In Tswana tradition both man and woman have a responsibility to be faithful. It was assumed that men tended toward infidelity and wives were counseled in the marriage ceremony itself to accept their husband's straying. The old saying was "A man, like a bull, cannot be confined in a *kraal* [corral]." The modern version now heard in discussions of faithfulness uses the two local staples of the diet—cornmeal and rice—to make the metaphor: "A man cannot live on *pap* all his life, but must sometimes have rice."

The infidelities of men and women were not treated as equally serious in the old culture, but a man did have a duty to care for his wife, including faithfulness in most situations. He could be punished for affairs.

What has gotten lost in the mix of Western and African culture is the punishment for unfaithfulness for husbands. Families are now fractured in time and space, and tribal authority to rein in the behavior of men has dissipated. The logic and cohesiveness of the culture has developed fissures. Now, this ancient version of "faithfulness" has become dangerous.

Roads in Africa are the streams that carry HIV—where the roads go, the virus can follow. When HIV first began to move in Africa, it was the trans-African highway from Kenya, through Uganda, to the Congo that carried this live cargo. It was hauled in the cabs of the trucks, inside the bodies of the drivers. They made stops and deposited swarms of particles along the way, from whence the virus spread to cities and rural areas surrounding the truck routes.

The image of the road describes not only the travel of the virus, but in another way describes its entrance into human society. Imagine rain falling on pavement. The water pools and does not break through, except where there are cracks in the surface. At those breaks the rain can penetrate, moving down and then spreading beneath the pavement. Once it is under the surface water compacts the grains of sand and dirt, eliminating pockets. The settling in some spots and not others means the roadway begins to waffle and crack. Potholes appear and edges of the roadway begin to shear off. The breakup of the entire road is underway.

So it is with HIV: As this particle rains down on humans, it seeks out the small breaks in culture. As families break and partners turn to others, a seam is opened. As people move from place to place, seeking comfort from other partners, the fissure opens. The undermining of society begins.

In science the couplings of love are sometimes expressed in mathematical models. They are like fluid flows, or combustion spreading.

When two people have a relationship, and one or the other occasionally strays, thereby introducing a third element to the movement of biological fluids, the risk begins. But if the unfaithfulness is not sustained over many encounters, the virus may remain trapped within the more or less faithful pair.

Add the extra partner on a regular basis, though, and the relationship basically becomes no longer two-way, but three- or four-way.

These openings among others in the "couples" become stable passages through which the virus can move.

In each individual sexual encounter the odds of passing the virus vary—from one time in fifty to one in ten thousand, depending on other things. (For example, for a period of three to six weeks after a person is first infected, the virus multiplies rapidly in the body, so tens to hundreds of thousands of viral particles are present in every milliliter of blood. Later in the infection the immune system is at work and the number of virus particles drops ten- to a hundredfold. Or, in another example, if a person has another sexually-transmitted disease, the sores from it greatly increase the chance of passing the virus.)

All this means that a steady diet of sex, say, three times per week, can make passing the virus a near certainty between two people over a year or two. Add the third party, and a great amplification of mathematical risk occurs.

Unfaithfulness exists in all cultures, but there are several different patterns. In some places, such as the United States and Europe, multiple sex partners are common, but mostly the partnerships are serial—people don't usually go with more than one partner at a time. This is referred to as "serial monogamy." In Asia a somewhat similar pattern exists, but with an emphasis on flings. Dalliances with other partners occur, but partners return to their main squeeze after short affairs. In these situations, HIV can be passed easily, but not so quickly.

Unfortunately, add a dollop of faith*ful*ness to the mix, and you have the pattern of stable but overlapping relationships common in southern Africa. In Botswana, polygamy is outlawed and infidelity is frowned upon. But at the same time, the traditional marriage ceremony still carries this counseling for the bride: Wives are advised that for a happy marriage it is important not to ask a husband where he has been at night. Loyalty is more important, lest a woman create mistrust. The same advice is not passed on to the groom.

Thus, Africans are caught in transition between two African values—faithfulness and male authority.

What has been learned from this collision of values has meaning for those who want to stop the HIV epidemic. It suggests that from a purely practical point of view the two warring factions who emphasize abstinence and faithfulness or condoms and knowledge have both been right in some ways.

Faithfulness is vital. But also, condoms can be very effective. And in both cases, knowledge and testing are indispensable.

In the three successful cases of prevention documented around the world—in Senegal, Thailand, and Uganda—there were two key factors. People reduced the number of partners they had, and increased their condom use. There are fancier ways of saying these things: "Be faithful" and "change your behavior" emphasize a different approach to loving, while "condomize" and "safe sex" emphasize practical precautions.

When the international team arrived to begin their challenge to AIDS in Botswana, they started with a plan that read precisely like something from a corporate office. What's needed? Computers, IT plans, counselors, doctors, trucks, refrigerators. How long it would take to bring them in? How long would the training take? How much it would cost?

It said that in Botswana, a nation of about 1.5 million people, something more than 300,000 adults were infected with HIV. They had calculated that not all were equally sick, but that about 110,000 of them were already in need of triple-drug treatment. The project would treat 19,000 the first year, and then ramp up to the full 110,000 over the next four years.

Some 108 new doctors, nurses, and pharmacists would be brought in. An array of new prefab clinic buildings would be put up. Training by experts would be provided for all the key people in Botswana's health system, from social workers to counselors and MDs. Condoms would be provided in the millions, both free and through discounted "social marketing" plans. Education would be brought in to the public schools from grade school to university. Market research, including focus groups and other polling methods, would be used to create the right messages and deliver them to the right citizens. The center of the system would be a computer network that would keep track of all patients, from the time they came forward for tests, all over the country on an instantaneous basis. That way, when a patient showed up at a clinic, his or her updated record would be in hand at any place.

The system was built to address the problems they expected to see: difficulty ensuring that patients took their medicines; effort needed to visit patients in their homes as well as waiting for them in the clinic; full counseling for the difficult problems of stigma; and effective public messages about HIV and the project itself.

The experts who worked in Botswana were completely unprepared for what they actually faced. If they had known, they probably would have first hired some experts on Botswana culture and begun with visits to tribal chiefs in the villages and bureaucrats in the city. They learned, of course, but it was a painful process with long, long delays.

While it was tough going, the project was something never really tried before, and it led the way in Africa. It did prove that critics were wrong about bringing sophisticated medicines to Africa; Africans take their medicine as well as or better than Westerners, and the drugs are just as effective as anywhere else, even considering that the patients coming in are sicker in Africa.

The obstacles were not the expected logistical difficulties—from watches to strict routines of medicine taking—but cultural, and the full array of expensive clinics, doctors, and nurses once thought to be essential could actually be a hindrance to delivering lifesaving treatment. The Botswana experiment lit up the path that other countries in Africa and Asia have now started following.

Donald de Korte, a Dutch doctor who had been Merck's managing director in South Africa for some years, was brought on to lead the grand experiment. He is a tall man, with sandy, gray-streaked hair and a ruddy complexion.

He became the director of what was named ACHAP, for the African Comprehensive HIV/AIDS Partnership. He is blunt, impatient with those not working to speed, but has a sense of humor about life and the difficulties ahead.

He looks like a man comfortable outdoors, and in one of his early adventures in Botswana he did head out into one of the wilderness parks in a four-wheel safari vehicle. He was soon halted by the tough driving—deep mud, to be exact—and it took two days for rescuers to reach him and haul him out.

He was confident, a game fellow.

De Korte was aware that the project was a risk, for Botswana, for Merck, and for himself personally because of the chance of failure. And after laying the ground for the plan for months, he had already encountered unexpected trouble.

De Korte found that there were widespread vacancies in Botswana's health staff—perhaps as many as 25 percent of the positions were unfilled. But the ministries that had failed to fill the jobs, the government now insisted, would also be in charge of recruiting the 108 new doctors, pharmacists, and nurses needed in the new program. De Korte asked to hire the 108 separately, fresh staff to work alongside current staff, rather than filling current holes in the system.

But as time went on, intransigence increased. The parallel staff was not only disapproved, but after de Korte had recruited dozens of doctors and nurses from other African countries, the usual process took over and destroyed recruitment.

The usual procedures—two interviews spaced months apart, approval by several ministries, finding funds from the treasury—would normally take a year and a half before a new hire could come to work. Needless to say, doctors in Africa, much in demand, cannot keep their lives and families on hold while waiting for consultations to be followed in careful order in Botswana. So in the second year of the program, more than forty prospective doctors had been recruited— and then were lost to the system because of delay.

It took two and a half years after the announcement of the program in Botswana to begin bringing doctors in. And when they arrived there were still disputes among government officials, and the doctors went for months without pay.

When it came to building a little prefabricated clinic on the grounds of the main hospital, Princess Marina in the capital, de Korte was told to allow the government to build it through the usual system. Eighteen months later nothing had been done. De Korte pleaded with the president himself, and was finally given power to build the clinic; it was up in less than three months.

The normal operation of the government was set by old cultural habits. The tribes had an unusually democratic way of governing themselves. They were led by chiefs, but all major decisions tradition- ally have been submitted to the whole population of the village. That meant meeting at the *kgotla*—a public space under a large tree where all villagers could assemble. At such meetings, which could last for days or weeks, each citizen was expected to speak his piece and debate the matter at hand. Then the chief would make a decision, usually based on what he felt the consensus was. This type of consultation be- fore decisions is a conservative mechanism that has served the tribes well for eight hundred years, keeping them stable and peaceful.

The principle is one of consultation (*therisanyo* in Setswana, one language used in Botswana). The dignity of each person in society is maintained by recognizing his position, as shown by the gesture to get his consent when a matter is at issue.

Translated into modern government, that means that many officials have the right to be heard from, and to give or withhold support for the measure going forward. The effect is of a system that is careful to follow rules and works well to weed out corruption and renegade decision makers.

The doctor hired to lead the toughest challenge, building the drug treatment program for the nation, was Ernest Darkoh. His family is from Ghana, but he was raised in Kenya and Tanzania, and then went to school in the United States. He earned his MD from Harvard, but felt that ordinary medicine really didn't address the larger problems of the world, so he decided to study public health. After gaining his MPH, he realized that the big problems in health all have major parts that are about management and money. So he took an MBA from Oxford. Then, to get real world experience, he took a job with the McKinsey consulting firm, well known for its work in health systems.

Eventually, he was asked to take on the challenge of Botswana.

When he arrived one of his first encounters was with the board appointed by the government to oversee the big project. He jumped in enthusiastically, talking about rolling out plans.

But he found that the government-appointed board had not been authorized to make any decisions. It was a board built, in the midst of a raging epidemic, to discuss matters. He was told the board had no mandate yet, could not hire or fire or make any lasting decisions.

"The sole reason for creating the team was to be empowered and to make decisions," Darkoh said, but in fact what was created was another layer of bureaucracy even before the work started. "It was literally very scary," he said. "This was not the way to run a national emergency. From the beginning it was ten steps forward, twelve steps back. You have major victories, and then the next day you're ready to pack up and go."

A central problem was also encouraging people to get HIV tests. Under the elaborate system developed on the American model, testing involved multiple trips and permissions and counseling, raising great barriers to getting lifesaving drugs to the people. The solution proposed was to change the whole approach to testing, removing the elaborate counseling sessions and visits, and creating rather a routine medical procedure done whenever a patient shows up at the hospital. Patients had the right to refuse, but if they didn't object, they would get HIV tests.

Darkoh said that the policy was controversial because it went against policies established over years in the West built to guarantee consent and confidentiality. It was built in the years when disclosure of infection would bring down stigma, alienation, and potential job loss. Because there had been no good treatments, and the government had not offered care to the sick, it had been clear that forced testing could have led to harm, and would have done little good for the infected.

But by the time the epidemic had swept Botswana, the situation had changed greatly. The stigma was still present, but the government was offering lifesaving drugs and full care, at no cost. And with more than a third of the whole nation infected, it was a vital state interest to find out who was infected and to try to treat them and counsel them not to spread the disease further. It was President Mogae who broke the jam over testing, and he pressed through the new "routine testing" policy.

Two years into the project the infrastructure was still being built, and the 19,000 patients treated in the first year turned out to be much less—3,200 after eighteen months, and most of that was done by a handful of doctors working absurd hours because manpower recruitment was still caught in the hands of multiple, slow decision makers.

By 2003, de Korte was frustrated and under great stress. He had become a customer for pharmaceuticals himself: He started on Prozac. Darkoh had been ready to resign more than once.

Eventually the friction got to be too much. The board relieved de Korte of command in the fall of 2003, in hopes that the conflicts had to do with de Korte's tough personality and demands for performance. Few of those watching thought much would have been done at all without de Korte's pressure. But to prevent a complete and public breakdown of the project, Merck and Gates took the prudent step of bringing in a manager from within Botswana, Tsetsele Fantan, who had been the manager of the HIV program at the nation's largest mine, was appointed director of the Merck-Gates project.

Harriet would have appeared stately if she were able to stand to her full height, but she was still a little weak. She has been on the new drugs only a short time. Less than four weeks before, she was on a pallet in a dark room at the back of her mother's house. She could not walk.

Most healthy people have immune system cell counts of about

1,000; hers were down to 35 and diving to zero. By contrast, her blood was swarming with more than 300,000 HIV particles per deciliter of blood, and that count was rising. Her medical counts, in any clinic around the world at the time, were the numbers of death.

She was ready for it. She said she could do nothing more for her children. She had stopped weeping over her youngest daughter who had HIV, as she didn't have even the moisture in her eyes to make tears.

But one afternoon a friend who worked at the hospital came by to get her. She brooked no arguments, but simply lifted Harriet up and with some help carried her to a car, and then into the hospital. She was given a round of tests, though she was semiconscious and barely cared.

Within weeks she regained her appetite both for food and life. She started to walk again. Reporters in the capital of Botswana were keeping count, and they said that Harriet was the fifth person in the entire nation to openly admit being infected.

On the other side of the coin was a schoolteacher from a village south of the capital who asked that reporters not use his name. He understood about the disease and how it was passed. He knew in looking over his last few years that he had taken risks with girlfriends. He suspected he might well have the virus. But when he faced the terrible moment of going to get tested he realized with crystal clarity what it was all about.

He knew that he would likely walk into the testing center as one person, relatively healthy and well liked, a young man with friends, a good job, and a family, and walk out of the center as a ghost, a man whose friends did not want to touch him, whose neighbors would turn away in the street. His job would be in danger. It was as if he were being asked to end his life as a human and become a monster, some kind of shamed creature, all voluntarily. Death didn't seem so serious a consequence compared to a life of being humiliated daily.

After many attempts and great pressure from his wife, he finally did get tested. But now that he knows he has the virus, he still keeps it a secret from his friends and the school where he works.

Botswana has no medical school, so all the Batswana who are doctors must go abroad for training. Not all come back, and among those who do, few ever went to work for the government. The pay is low and there has been little effort to recruit them. It is a significant loss for the country.

Ndwapi Ndwapi, born in a village in northern Botswana and schooled in the capital, spent ten years being trained in medicine in the United States. When he came back his training was perfect— infectious diseases—for him to be grabbed up by his nation's emergency AIDS program.

He is a tall young man with round cheeks and a small mustache. His gaze is intense. When he speaks he sounds like a man in the trenches, under constant fire. He is now head of the largest HIV clinic in Botswana, in the hospital in the capital. He had had to fight his own government to get there.

When he arrived back from his training in the United States, he says, "They were very glad to see me" at the ministry of health. But they took some months before giving him an assignment; they wanted him to take his place at the bottom of the ladder in Botswana—a posting in a low-ranking job two hundred miles from the capital at a salary of about $2,500 per year. He could have earned about $120,000 to start in the United States and could have moved quickly into his specialty; accounting for cost of living differences, a $30,000 salary would be expected in Botswana.

"It's completely nuts," he says, "and it's symptomatic of the system."

Having left and come back, he can see Botswana in the light of other ways of doing things. So his first response to his treatment when he returned was anger and frustration. He was in some ways in the same position as the outsiders from ACHAP who were fighting to make things happen on an emergency basis. He had to battle for his job in an AIDS program even though it was desperately short of doctors, especially doctors who understood Batswana culture and language.

He says, frustrated as he was, that he understood where the slowness came from. Now that he was back he felt it was his duty to help change the dysfunctional things about the slow system in Botswana.

It is a cultural inheritance with a distinguished past now caught in an emergency that makes it break down.

In emergencies, it fails, says Ndwapi. "The money's there, the will is there, the know-how is there, but somehow, you can't hire the people you want to hire. We know for a fact that there are doctors throughout Africa and other places in the world that would love to do this job. And yet, somehow, it just doesn't happen," he says.

To protest, to fight the dignified system of respect and consultation is considered shameful, putting your personal interests above the good of the group. But Ndwapi began to argue loudly for quick decision making, and for bypassing some usual procedures. "I was more than willing, and I still am more than willing, to take responsibility for whatever happens," he says, "for whatever comes down on my head.

"If I make decisions on my own sometimes, I can sleep at night because I know that the alternative is a hundred times worse than anything I can do. The alternative is doing nothing."

As we sat in a tiny cubicle at the Princess Marina Hospital, near a long corridor lined on both sides by patients who have been waiting for several hours, he says that the war on HIV must come down to this, in some ways, everywhere: fighting to make a system not set up to handle health emergencies take them on aggressively.

He mentions the prefab clinic that had been the subject of fights between ACHAP and the government. It was finally built, he says, "but you know it's not being used yet."

"Why?"

"Because there are no phones. Because there is no paper. In Botswana, we run out of paper." There is money to buy paper, but it doesn't get bought and delivered. The supply office refers to the ministry that controls procurement, and that ministry refers to another ministry, which says it has not sent supply money because it's been asked to close its books to end the fiscal period by another ministry. When you get to the ministry of finance, they say the folks are wrong, they are still supposed to be buying paper.

"You see what I mean?"

But on a day in May 2003, the prefab clinic does, finally, open for business. Gradually, changes happen. Slowly, new ways of doing things are installed.

Ndwapi is a man struggling to push his culture forward much

faster than it wants to go. In the face of years of success that suggests the culture has done well, he must argue that it is now stumbling. It is a struggle not just for the lives of those in the hallway, but for the future of the country, and for a way nations can work together.

It's tough, there are fights and suspicions, but it is the best way to do it, Ndwapi says. "The best way is to bring in an organization like ACHAP. Charge it with the responsibility of doing this, okay? And just give them the mission of setting it up and then integrating it into this nation." They must start it, hire and train local people, and then turn it over, he says. "Any time in the past two years we got anything significant done, it was because ACHAP has been involved. They took charge."

By 2004, the original leader, Donald de Korte was gone, and Darkoh and Ndwapi were beleaguered, but the fights had begun to pay off. All of the clinics envisioned in the original plan were finally up and running, albeit three years late. After the decision to make testing easier, those infected began coming forward in larger and larger numbers.

"We're going to take off," Ndwapi says. "This is beginning to work. You know, this is a country that is good with the big things. The little things on the ground are not so good, but the big things, knowing which way to go, we get those right."

The program did take off, finally. The number of people who were tested, enrolled in regular AIDS care, and getting the HIV drugs rose from 3,000 in early 2003, to 20,000 in mid 2004, to 43,000 by early 2005, and it is still rising.

The project has now surpassed all other African and Asian countries in its delivery of HIV care and drugs. Following Botswana's lead, twelve other African nations have now started bringing drug treatment to their HIV-infected citizens, and this time in Africa has been dubbed "the decade of treatment" for Africa, when the world's drugs and expertise finally began to turn to those who need them most.

A United Nations project called "3 by 5," has begun working toward the goal of treating three million people in the poor countries with top-end AIDS drugs by the end of 2005. The goal will not be met, but the pressure is on, and it is estimated that one million or more HIV-infected people in poor countries will be under treatment by that date.

Ernest Darkoh, after three years before the mast in Botswana, now says that there are strong lessons for others to follow when delivering AIDS drugs to poor countries. First, don't expect to see results quickly; development is not linear, it takes time to build up and learn what the real problems are before it takes off. Second, though it is natural to think of bringing on a treatment program slowly, beginning with central clinics in the capital, it is a mistake. The sickest patients come forward first, and because they need ten times more help than others, they overwhelm the system. There is also little to be gained from a slow scale-up—the problems at each new village clinic are the same as the previous ones, and must be learned anew at each place. So, he says, go for it. Scale up quickly, go to the rural areas nearest the patients' homes all at once. Then, bring in experts to work in each place for six months to train those who will have to take over.

Another lesson: Make testing as easy as possible, because you need to get to patients before they are at their sickest, and they can be better treated and returned to work the earlier they come in.

The final message is that "patients will spend ninety-nine percent of their lives in their communities, not at a hospital or a health facility."

Therefore, it is possibly wasteful and dangerous to emphasize the building of a "brick-and-mortar health care infrastructure." In fact, drugs can be delivered from the back of a truck if need be. But the vital job is to track the patients and their conditions.

"Therefore," says Darkoh, "for any new program, the highest priority and the bulk of the initial effort should go toward establishing a robust and reliable patient-tracking, monitoring, and evaluation system," with or without walls.

Along the way, the data from Botswana have proved skeptics wrong—Africans actually take their medicines much better than Westerners. On average, Africans take 90 percent of all their pills, compared to Americans, who take about 70 percent of their prescribed dose. In addition, in testing verbal reports, researchers found that Africans are more truthful when telling how many pills they missed compared to Americans. The Africans overestimate by 3 percent, whereas Americans overestimate their compliancy by 20 percent.

The cost of treating the Batswana, even though it was the first program and emphasized the need for high-level training and fully qualified doctors and nurses, cost about one-tenth or less than treatment in the United States. In Botswana treatment cost has so far ranged from $580 to $1,580 per person for a year. The cost is expected to drop considerably in coming years.

To come back to the patients themselves: Harriet, one of the first to get the drugs, within weeks of beginning treatment went to work as a volunteer, counseling other infected women. Eventually she got a paid job and became one of the top counselors. By the end of 2003 she was engaged to be married. Her life was beginning again.

And in the village of Molepolole, I visited Edwin Moses. He works as a consultant on a radio drama that tells stories of village life, including about AIDS.

On the road out of Gaborone, you turn at the filling station and then veer right toward the Kalahari Desert. There is a track that threads little fenced-in plots with their characteristic yards—no grass, but the reddish dirt has been carefully tidied by raking.

Two of Edwin's neighbors died of HIV recently, one from an infection triggered by the virus and another from suicide.

Edwin comes out of the concrete-block house, greeting me with a shy smile and a charming giggle. He is fundamentally a happy guy—never mind his circumstances.

He is infected with HIV. But his beaming face is also the new face of the epidemic in southern Africa. Edwin and people like him represent the beginning of a tide moving the other way. After he became infected and his infant son died, he began to change his life. He stayed away from women for a time, then hitched up with a woman from his village who was also infected, and also wary of love.

But together the two thought it through, and decided to marry. They are both healthy now, but they are tested and monitored regularly, and are ready to take the drugs when it's best for them to start. They even got a little plot of land, and are building a house.

Then they went the final step. They had a baby, and because medicine can now keep babies free of virus, she is negative. She has a future.

Edwin says he looks forward to telling little Virginia (named after the friend who brought him and his wife, Mariah, together) their story. "It will be a treasure to her," he said. The baby, ten months old, is making squawking noises and cooing sounds as we speak. She is non-chalantly standing with one hand on her mother's knee.

"She will know all about how it happened, how she was born, and knowing everything, it will make her free. It will be a great treasure. We are living for her now."

Edwin goes to funerals every weekend, but now he asks to speak for a few minutes, to suggest that people get themselves tested for the virus, so they can get help and treatment when the time comes. AIDS no longer means death, he says, we can live with it.

The feeling among those who have worked in Botswana on AIDS is a double sense that it is the hardest and most patience-consuming work they have ever done. They also feel that building programs here, with tens of thousands now getting regular high-level care, is an extraordinary achievement. The work is pioneering and should make the way somewhat easier, at least, as new programs are now built across Africa.

From Botswana and from each of the other successes I have described, there are fundamentals to be learned about the new "smart aid" approach.

First, in each case, there was strong leadership present—Fazle Abed and his coworkers at BRAC in Bangladesh, Ram Shrestha and his colleagues in Nepal, David Heymann and the polio team in India and elsewhere, and the combination of President Festus Mogae and the team at the African Comprehensive HIV/AIDS Partnership in Botswana. This does not exhaust the list of leaders on these projects, for good leaders tend to attract others who are effective. In each of these stories, one of the key issues leaders emphasize is a commitment to get results no matter what the obstacles or number of years it takes.

These leaders believe there is simply nothing more important for their nations than to deliver on this work. There can be no higher ambition than to make them succeed even if the work is hard and requires many tries to get each part of the project right. Blunders were made in each case, as I hope I have spelled out.

A further feature in common is that in three cases, the work was accomplished with inexpensive medicine and local volunteers. The fourth case, Botswana, used medicine that is not so cheap but still is a bargain relative to its cost in the developed nations. In each case, there is a high health impact for the money spent.

One thing that is vital is that scientific research was used effectively, coupled with good management, in each instance. None of these results would have been possible without scientific experiments showing what was effective, because people in the past have often made reasonable but quite incorrect guesses about what works in health. Scientific backup is indispensible.

Some of this is not obvious. We thought we knew a great deal about vitamin A, how the body uses it, what its chemistry is, and so forth. When scientists did the research, they discovered that we knew nothing about the single most vital fact about this body chemical. In Bangladesh, Fazle Abed, after three decades of work in the villages, has found that no matter how well he thought he knew the culture and how to get people organized, he didn't really know until he tried. In that regard, development is like science—it requires actual experimentation, data collection, and analysis to get things done, even when it's assumed things work a specific way. A good case in point is the topic of maternal mortality and infant mortality during the day of birth; in Western countries we think we know what's important for health at birth. But we have been wrong. We are just now discovering how to deliver babies with high success rates. For example, we know that germs can cause infection for both mother and baby at birth, but our Western solution has been a kind of blanket hygiene of the entire birth enviroment. However, in most places that is not possible. So now we must find out what the important parts of hygiene at birth are. Is it clean hands for the birth attendant? In many countries, probably not, because the midwives do not examine and handle mothers and babies in the intrusive way we do in most developed nations; the chances of infection are smaller from that route. But it turns out that how and when the cord is cut might be vital. Or putting the baby to the mother's breast immediately—not common in medical settings—may save many infants from dying due to lack of warmth or early nutrition. In new settings, we need new science.

The good management part of any project should go without saying, as successful work in any field requires it. In delivering aid it is important to keep in mind that culture is critical, and so local workers and a sense of local values must be present.

Another point worth making is that each project went forward with explicit plans to build up local infrastructure and systems for the long haul. Good programs don't come and go; they come and stay. This is one reason why they are so cost-effective.

The best practitioners say the essence of successful development is a humility before challenging work and a commitment to learn what is the right thing to do—not in general, but in this intervention, in this week or month. The other important factors—science, monitoring, management, cautious spending—all follow from this.

PART TWO

Meeting
the
Challenge

5

The Forgotten Link Between Health and Wealth

Whether the country is Botswana or Nepal, India or Bangladesh, there is much that can be effectively done to raise the level of health and with it, hope.

There is no shortage of skeptics on this topic. Some say that it is not our job to help our neighbors; they should help themselves. Others argue it will cost too much or be too difficult to carry it off properly. The skepticism flourishes, and the poor have few advocates.

Nevertheless, the first difficult steps have been taken. Nations have officially agreed to the idea of more than doubling aid when they signed on to the Millennium Development Goals and the Millennium Development Project. A couple of funding mechanisms have been started with the Global Fund to Fight AIDS, Tuberculosis and Malaria and President Bush's Millennium Challenge Account.

Now, the problem will be building the political support for an increase in aid that will meet the basic development needs of the poorest nations. It will cost about $50 billion beyond existing commitments.

But the dollar cost is not the hard part, it is building up the nerve to make such a commitment that is difficult. This reluctance is nothing new.

Government, said Adam Smith, has only three main duties: to provide for defense; to dispense justice; and to build necessary public works. It's the third that's always been a hard sell. As we confront the challenge of today's global health problems we would do well to consider the hard-earned lessons of the reformers who pioneered the modern notion that spending the public's money on disease prevention was not only the best moral course but the expedient course as well. It took four waves of epidemic cholera in England, which killed more than 120 million, and years of work by enlightened researchers to convince politicians in nineteenth-century Britain that health was, in fact, a public matter worth spending money on.

In the end, what was achieved was the Public Health Act and other laws that made possible the building of the London sewer and clean water system, the first of its kind and a model for the world. It was expensive—on the scale of the Marshall Plan after World War II—one of those rare moments of large but farsighted expenditure. The building of the system stopped the waves of cholera in England even as they continued to roil the cities of Europe that didn't build water and sewer systems. It also defused widespread protests about living conditions that had beset Britain as the extraordinary social changes, and dislocations, of that first great globalization of the world's economy heated up.

Historian R. A. Lewis, who chronicled the rise of the public health movement, wrote that the greatest obstacle that had to be overcome in the campaign was not, as might have been expected, anti-government spending conservatism per se, because in fact many conservatives understood the value of the investment; rather it was a kind of conservatism "which is blind to the benefits of the simplest improvements." The story of England's defeat of cholera is just one of such simple improvements—simple approaches much like those profiled in the preceeding chapters—supported by a movement of large ambition; just the sort of mobilization of public will and resources that we need today. The story is also a cautionary tale about the dangers of forgetting the vital link between health and wealth, and is relevant to the issue of what has gone wrong for so many years with foreign aid programs that did in fact forget that link.

The port of Sunderland was one of the biggest in England in 1831, one of the boom towns of the nineteenth-century globalization. As more and more goods flowed in and out of the port a crush of people flooded the town looking for work. But wages were low and housing scant, and thousands were pressed into filthy dockside neighborhoods with no sewers, ventilation, or ready supplies of clean water.

In September and October many ships came into port from Hamburg and Riga on the Baltic Sea. Doctors in Sunderland had read the news from those ports: All summer outbreaks of Asiatic cholera had wracked Russia's and Germany's shores. The disease had swept up from India the previous year, moving through Alexandria and Constantinople, then to the Caspian Sea, finally reaching the Russian army. Reports said that troops in Poland and Germany had set up cordons sanitaire, but they failed to keep the cholera at bay, and so by September the disease had infiltrated both Riga and Hamburg—from which the ships lying in Sunderland harbor had just departed. Cholera had never been in England or Europe before, and the doctors in town knew little about cholera beyond its name.

Then late on a Sunday night, the sixteenth of October, Ellen Isabella Hazard, a girl living in the slums around Sunderland's wharf on Low Street, woke up terribly ill. She was described in news accounts as a common girl, but her death was anything but common. Her symptoms seemed to clearly fit the description of Asiatic cholera.

This new disease was unlike the familiar forms of death of the century. Tuberculosis was so well known that it had even been romanticized in literature, with characters bravely facing death through TB's slow passage from health, through paleness, to disappearance. Cholera, in contrast, came on suddenly and with furious force. It is, in fact, among the fastest-acting killer diseases known. Its symptoms begin with a vague feeling of queasiness, and within only hours advance to the most painful spasms of the gut, soon followed by retching and the loss of half the body's water. Within a day's time the constant flushing of the system leads to acute dehydration—a lack of water and oxygen—and the sufferer takes on the pinched, blue cast of choleric death. "To see individuals well in the morning and buried before night, retiring apparently well, and dead in the morning, is something which is appalling to the boldest heart," one patient wrote. Half of those who came down with the illness during this epidemic were killed by it.

Sunderland doctors William Clanny and James Kell were sure that

Ellen Hazard had died of the Asiatic cholera. Kell had seen the symptoms of the disease once when he was traveling in the Indian Ocean. He argued to town officials that a quarantine of the ships coming into the harbor was essential. The quarantine was ordered on November 1, and a British frigate was sent to close the port. The business life of the town was frozen.

But as in Riga and Hamburg the plague had already found a foothold. Describing the effects it soon reaped, Clanny wrote that he had never seen Sunderland in such a state of filth among crowded neighborhoods filled with all those who had recently come looking for work: "It appeared to us that the atmosphere carried pestilence with it, as several persons were as suddenly affected by it as if they had been struck by lightning."

Yet, even as conditions grew grimmer, the local businessmen were not willing to accept the quarantine, and organized a revolt. Drawing together doctors who had never seen victims of the cholera from Asia, the businessmen soon met en masse and declared that Sunderland was as healthy as it had ever been. They issued a statement saying this was no epidemic but merely a few cases. Further, they declared, the disease was "not the Indian Cholera, or of any foreign origin." Those who had died had been stricken with common bowel problems "which visited every town in the kingdom in the autumn," they asserted, "aggravated by want and uncleanliness."

Under the pressure, the town board reversed its position and the quarantine was called off. The plague was unleashed to spread at will.

By January, 215 deaths had been reported in Sunderland, and many more in towns nearby. The disease soon moved to Newcastle, and by

February reached London and Edinburgh. By spring, in the first eighteen days of the epidemic in Paris, 7,000 were dead. In England, by the end of the summer more than 20,000 had succumbed.

This was the world's first truly global epidemic, extending finally from New Delhi to New York, Singapore to San Francisco. The epidemic of 1832 was, in addition, just the first of five great waves of cholera to come in the nineteenth century.

The voracious spread of cholera is a striking case in point of the way that disease outbreaks often follow globalization. "Once it had arrived," wrote historian Richard J. Evans, "it fastened on to the industrial society that was then in the making and exploited and exaggerated many of its most prominent aspects, from urbanization and overcrowding to environmental pollution and social inequality." Though it was not the greatest killer of the time—the nineteenth century was the age of epidemics—the fact that it was an invasion from a foreign country was feared and resented. It also came just as conditions in society worsened. These things made it the signature disease of its day. One doctor of the time recalled, "Our other plagues were home-bred, and part of ourselves, as it were; we had a habit of looking at them with a fatal indifference, indeed, in as much as it led us to believe that they could be effectually subdued. But the cholera was something outlandish, unknown, monstrous."

When the cholera epidemics began there were no public health boards in England, Europe, or America. By the end of the epidemics all the major countries had them. At the beginning, governments did not have the power to clean up streets, sewers, and water supplies; by the end, each large nation had established public bodies to seize the initiative and punish those causing needless filth and disease. This achievement did not, however, come easily.

Then, as now, many objections to the government playing an active role in public welfare, and especially to spending public money on those efforts, were raised.

A cadre of intellectuals, clergymen, and misfits came together to advocate for workers and the poor. They discovered the key insights and did the legwork needed to put public health on the agenda in nineteenth-century England. One such dogged visionary was Englishman Edwin Chadwick, a journalist and lawyer who was too low-born to ever gain a government title. He became something of a freelance advocate attached to one commission after another investigating social problems. He created the first well-documented social exposé, a powerful study that became the most influential single work in the creation of public health. Entitled "An Inquiry into the Sanitary Conditions of the Labouring Population of Great Britain," the report laid out the suffering and death caused by the filthy state of the towns, with their open sewers, contaminated wells, and shabby, ill-heated housing crammed with six to ten persons per room. He conducted hundreds of interviews, compiled masses of statistics, and made charts and graphs that were powerful in their effect, disproving the popular notions of the time about the laziness of workers, that the poor were themselves responsible for their lot. He identified the important factors on which a new economy could begin to build—those that would keep the workers well-nourished and in good health.

History has had difficulty classifying Edwin Chadwick. He was a conservative, but a social reformer as well. He dedicated his adult life to efforts to improve the lot of working people, but kept his reforms inside the bounds of capitalist thinking. In some ways he avoided taking on the fundamental issues of poverty and inequality.

Chadwick looked benign, with large, liquid eyes and a round, affable walrus face. In person, he didn't seem fearsome, but in his era, the 1830s to the 1860s, Edwin Chadwick became the most hated man in England: He was the man who had dreamed up the terrible workhouses for the poor that Charles Dickens brought to such horrifying life in depicting the worst of nineteenth-century existence. Yet, by the end of his career, Chadwick was also counted as the man who did more for the common people's health and well-being in England than any other single person in the long, tumultuous nineteenth century.

Chadwick thought the best way to increase the nation's wealth was by supplying industry with productive workers—good for business, good for workers. He believed in Adam Smith's dictum that economies must be driven by the engine of the free market, and he was aware that he was witnessing the creation of the first great industrial economy in England, the first booming success of capitalism. He was also confident that the economic boom would spread to all parts of the earth within the next century. But he perceived that at the heart of the engine there was a potentially hobbling problem. Working men and women were being pushed into terrible, unhealthy conditions.

A new field of knowledge was being created at the time that Chadwick thought could help solve this problem. It was referred to as "political arithmetic" because it used details from large numbers of people to outline problems. (The name has changed to statistics, from numbers for the "state.") He realized that numerical counts often contradicted our fondest delusions and led to keen insights.

In the spirit of the new statistics Chadwick launched a full-scale survey of the nation, the first of its kind, to describe the exact conditions of housing, water, sewage, health, sickness, and death among the working people of every district. The labor took three years. When the survey report was finished Chadwick put it before the Poor Law's board of commissioners. They were deeply shocked and could not bring themselves to publish it. The report was not only a huge compendium of horribles, but it contained the *names* of landlords and the corrupt private water and sewer boards. They knew that Chadwick would not sit still if they killed the report, so they simply disowned it. "We shall present it as *his* report, without making ourselves responsible for it," said the head of the board, George Lewis. Chadwick published it under his own name.

In the report, Chadwick produced one startling chart on the average age at death. Professionals of one district were listed in one column and laborers from the same district in another. In Derby, the average age at death for professionals was forty-nine; for laborers, twenty-one. In Bethnal Green, which housed some of the worst slums, professionals died on average at forty-five and workers at sixteen. Chadwick pointed out that the laborers who died were generally living above the level of subsistence. What they did not have was any of the vital services—clean water and sanitary ways to dispose of waste. Chadwick illustrated these tables with "sanitary maps" of Bethnal Green and Liverpool, which showed black crosses for deaths and how they were heavily concentrated in the filthiest districts.

Poverty, he showed, was not the *cause* of sicknesses; the causal logic ran in the reverse. Once a worker got sick the deepest poverty and trouble followed. He estimated that of those families receiving relief money in 1840, about 70 percent to 80 percent had lost their breadwinner to infectious diseases that could have been prevented with basic sanitation.

The whole difficulty, he said, came down to one of mental effort, of the will to understand the situation. The problem was relatively easy to address. Where some form of sewers already existed, as an example, he explained that the solution to this problem was just a matter of using the right materials to turn them from stagnant to flowing. Sewers had been essentially trenches, or brick-lined tunnels, that easily clogged or collapsed; he just asked engineers what would work better, and they told him: smooth, oval-shaped pipes, set on grades so water and debris would flow smoothly down. It worked.

Simple solutions could be effective, and must be put in place. If the situation were ignored, government was in effect turning over the towns of England to a group of people living in terrible conditions who were likely to end up at the torchlight protests of the time, and who were susceptible to radical ideas that "threaten the established order."

As biographer R. A. Lewis put it, "Chadwick drew his respectable hearers to the edge of the pit, and bade them observe the monsters they were breeding beneath their feet." The report was issued on July 9, 1842, and became an immediate bestseller.

Even as Chadwick's report was popularizing his argument for government's provision of a basic sanitation system in all neighborhoods, cholera was striking once again. Quiet since the first epidemic of 1831, in 1848 it came sweeping back across Britain. It arrived in Scotland, imported probably from Asia via the Baltic again, and over the years 1848 and 1849 the dead were counted at more than 53,000. Tens of thousands also perished in Europe as part of this epidemic. The political arithmetic that Chadwick and others had begun to apply to the life and death of British citizens was now taken a step further by another of the most influential public health innovators, a London doctor named John Snow. The simple solution he devised to a local outbreak of the epidemic, in his own neighborhood, has gone down in the annals of the history of public health, yet its powerful lesson has been forgotten by too many health advocates through the years.

Snow was a mild man with the great muttonchops popular in his day, matched to thinning locks combed over the top of his balding pate. He was a shy, quirky figure, and an unconvincing speaker. But he ran a thriving practice in London and was the celebrated creator of the new use of chloroform as an anesthetic. In fact, he gave the stuff to Queen Elizabeth to ease the pain of her eighth delivery, of Prince Leopold in 1853. He had also been one of the doctors called north to treat the ill in the cholera epidemic of 1831, and when the next wave hit London sixteen years later, it arrived in his own Soho neighborhood.

There was still great mystery about this sudden killer and why it appeared and disappeared. At the beginning of one of the waves of epidemic the medical journal *The Lancet* published an editorial laying out the frustration of doctors: "The question, What is cholera? is left unsolved."

Snow began researching the source of cholera, doubting the popular theory that the air carried the disease. He himself had seen that the disease attacked the gut, not the lungs.

Undertaking a series of investigations of the link between contaminated water and cholera, his first discovery was that there were more cholera deaths in a London district that had less sanitary water than in one with cleaner water. He published the result in a scientific paper, but he realized that this would not be enough to convince doubters. One doctor quickly pointed out that it could be the air in the two London locales that mattered, not the feces-polluted water. The chief statistician who kept the nation's new register, William Farr, was interested in Snow's theory, but dubious. A more powerful experiment would be needed, he said, to prove Snow's correlation. Such an experiment seemed impossible, however.

As it happened, conditions for a grand natural experiment *did* exist in London. Parliament had previously told water companies to move their pipes that took in "fresh" water so that these pipes were upstream of London, where water sources were less polluted. One water company had failed to do so, while another in the same area had quickly moved their pipes to cleaner sources. Many streets in London were supplied by both companies—the Lambeth Waterworks Company and the Southwark and Vauxhall Water Company—and they were competing pipe for pipe.

All Snow needed to do was go to the houses where cholera death occurred and check which company supplied the house. Was it the water from the pipes originating in London, and therefore less sanitary, or from the other pipes? By the end of 1853, from preliminary numbers, Snow had the answer. In districts supplied by Southwark there were 114 deaths per 10,000 people. In districts supplied about equally by both companies, there were 60 deaths per 10,000. And in the area supplied only by Lambeth with upstream water, there were no deaths recorded. The results were powerful.

But Snow didn't stop there. He pressed ahead with a study in his own neighborhood. People there were confident that yet a new epidemic of cholera which hit in 1854 would pass them by. The two previous epidemics had taken little toll there, and the water supplied was believed to be good, especially from the pump in Broad Street near Golden Square.

Yet death came, with the first occurring on the first day of September. By the third of September there was talk of an outbreak of cholera beginning in Golden Square, and by Saturday a yellow flag had been posted at the corner to warn strangers that disease had come.

Snow went house to house investigating and found that the first victim had apparently been an infant whose diapers had been dumped into the cesspool beside the Broad Street pump. Within days people for blocks all around had fallen ill.

Snow then went to the office of the General Register and looked up deaths by neighborhood. On Thursday, there were four deaths in the houses along the three blocks of Broad Street near its water pump. On Friday and Saturday there were seventy-nine deaths in the same stretch. He measured out the distances from house to pump, and then measured the distance to the next nearest pump in each direction. Seventy-three of the eighty-three dead lived closer to the Broad Street pump than to any other water pump. He went through the neighborhood, door to door, and inquired about who had used the pump and when. A brewery in the neighborhood was spared any deaths; they drank only beer at work. But a small factory nearby that drew water from the pump lost half its employees.

On the afternoon of September 7 Snow approached the parish board and told them the pump was most probably the source of disease. He suggested a profoundly simple and completely cost-free solution: removing the pump handle. The board was dubious but did as he asked, by way of an experiment. A man was sent out the next day, Friday, to take off the handle. From that day, the epidemic in Broad Street dropped off dramatically.

Gradually, the rallying point for the reformers became a project to build a system in London that would provide clean water and carry off sewage—all of it out of sight beneath the streets. All their arguments about health and injustice and barriers to getting people to work productively came down to a push for the sewer project. The discoveries of Chadwick and Snow were impressive, but there remained substantial resistance in the government and among the wealthier population. Often it takes one final crisis, one unexpected episode, to open the chute for reform. That came with the weather in the summer of 1858. That summer the river levels sank, and sewage muck encrusted on the exposed banks. In the heat, a great stench arose from the banks.

Suddenly, the houses of Parliament overlooking the river no longer found themselves at a comfortable distance from the problem of London's foul waters. They could not tolerate the stink, and at first ordered deodorants to be spread around and cloths saturated with chloride of lime as a disinfectant to be hung in the windows. But all efforts failed. Parliament, finally, was evacuated "by the sheer force of the stench" and moved upstream to reassemble.

The summer of 1858 is now called the summer of "the Great Stink." British prime minister Benjamin Disraeli, despite his lack of interest in spending money on any public service, felt forced to support the sewer and water project, which would be constructed under the Public Health Law passed ten years before but not acted on. Chadwick by this time had been forcibly retired, and Snow died just as the sewer vote was being taken. But the project went forward.

The great London sewer system was completed in 1870, with fixes to assure that all household and sewage water was either filtered or had no way to reenter the water system. One thousand miles of street sewers were built along with eighty-two miles of interceptors—innovative egg-shaped pipes that prevented clogs and seepage at corners or joints. It was the largest public works project in history at the time. The total cost was about £80 million, the equivalent in current dollars of more than the entire annual budget of the United States. The investment was well worth it: The cholera epidemics ceased, and London set the sanitation standard for the world.

The line from the entry of cholera into England and the home of Ellen Hazard, through the efforts of Chadwick and Snow, to the concrete solution of the new sewer system may not have been straight, but it was a single bright thread that could be followed, and it was in country after country around the world. Parallel developments took place in each of the leading developed countries of the nineteenth century. Cholera broke out, political turmoil ensued, and agitation for reform led to public health laws entailing many new government duties. The story powerfully demonstrates that on some matters of health only government action on a large scale is effective. The achievement was less than some wanted, but nonetheless this was a success of a kind never accomplished before—a real reduction in sickness and death for most people in the society.

The fact that the improvements in health that arose from the Public Health Act and its parallels in other countries marked the beginning of a new round of growing prosperity only became clear many years later. It was part of the economic boom of the last quarter of the nineteenth century in England, the richest time that nation had seen. It was also a milestone in the building of the vital revolution around the world—the rise of public health measures and disease prevention, both in research and in policy, from which we still benefit.

Unfortunately, the vital link between basic disease prevention and economic development was deemphasized during the post–World War II period, when a new theory of economic development, and a new regime of foreign aid programs, rose to prominence.

The effort to promote world economic development after World War II began well enough, at a United Nations financial conference held in July 1944 at Breton Woods, New Hampshire. The job was to rebuild Europe first, and then to save the world from future economic depressions. Two organizations were created for the task—the World Bank and the International Monetary Fund, which used aid and international cooperation to spur development. But at the time, funding for health projects was not at the top of the agenda.

The IMF was given the job of preventing another depression by keeping countries up to speed economically. To keep the world economy rolling, the conferees agreed, nations need to produce their fair share of demand and avoid letting their economies fall into slumps. The IMF would provide loans to those countries facing downturns, as well as advice about the best ways to spend the money to spur economic development. This was a recognition, wrote economist Joseph Stiglitz, that markets do not always work well, and thus there was a need for collective action at the global level for economic stability, just as the United Nations would provide collective action at a global level for political stability. The World Bank was created to aid in reconstructing Europe, but soon its primary mission shifted to giving development aid to poor countries.

These efforts to stimulate development were unprecedented in scale, and they were driven by a new theory of economic growth put forward, famously, by historian and economist Walt Whitman Rostow, in his highly influential book *The Stages of Economic Growth: A Non-Communist Manifesto.*

The key idea for building up poor countries was that growth came primarily from capital investments. If a country is to grow, it must have large amounts of money available to invest in business, roads, harbors, machinery. So the leading economic powers must become donors, it was suggested, who would supply the difference to the poor nations between the resources they had available for such investment and the amount deemed necessary to generate approximately 5 percent growth per year. The money would be provided in the form of low-interest, long-term loans.

"What I am talking about," Rostow wrote in a preface to a later edition,

> *is the third conscious attempt to provide for the human race by common endeavor a framework of stable peace, human freedom, and reasonable levels of economic welfare. The first two such efforts failed, the First World War yielding the Second, and the Second giving way to a protracted and distorting, if somewhat less bloody, cold war. But the Covenant of the League of Nations and the Charter of the United Nations both captured quite adequately the abiding aspirations of the people. And so we must try again.* The Stages of Economic Growth *thus suggests that the end of this millennium is not the end of history but rather a time to resume a quest we cannot abandon.*

Fundamental to his theory was the contention that all nations could naturally rise up from poverty with sufficient capital, and he said that there were several stages of growth through which societies passed, from the traditional society in which each generation is like the one before and advancement is not expected, all the way to the mature, growing industrial society. Economic growth, he argued, is a matter of natural evolution, like the natural evolution in human society from the struggle for mere survival to a higher form of society with a devotion to freedom and spirituality.

International stability did materialize in the postwar years, though that stability was due at least as much to the rigorously managed spheres of power presided over by the United States and the Soviet Union in the cold war as to economic development. Most of the poor nations failed to thrive, and the experts had to concede that spurring development was much harder than Rostow's theory had suggested. "The quest for a theory of growth and development has tormented us economists," wrote economist William Easterly, "as long as there have been economists." After more than fifty years of efforts the post–World War II approach to foreign aid has become the subject of raging debate about whether aid has had much effect at all on the well-being in poorer countries.

Foreign aid has become such a grab bag of different kinds of money given for different reasons that it is quite difficult to analyze, which hasn't helped settle the debate. Well-placed aid for development certainly seems to have helped a number of countries, such as South Korea, Taiwan, Uganda, and Mozambique. Overall in the past several decades, each dollar of aid targeted to growth added about $1.64 to the recipient's incomes, wrote economist Steven Radelet in *Foreign Policy* magazine. Aid targeted to health has done still better. But, he said, it has not been enough to have the needed effects in creating newly prosperous nations and turning poor nations toward the kind of aspirations for wealth and democracy that Americans have.

The standing complaints about foreign aid over the years have been that the money is applied like a balm, often without clear goals. It is given too often to governments that are corrupt or badly organized, so money may be either stolen or wasted. It has been given out by donor groups that decide how it should be spent—too often serving the interests of the donor rather than the recipient in need.

Martin Wolf, now chief economic writer for the *Financial Times* and a senior economist at the World Bank in the 1970s, said his experience of aid was bitter:

> *By the late 1970s, I had concluded that for all the good intentions and abilities of its staff, the Bank was a fatally flawed institution. The most important source of its failures was its commitment to lending, almost regardless of what was happening in the country it was lending to. This was an inevitable flaw since the institution could hardly admit that what it had to offer—money— would often make little difference. But this flaw was magnified by the personality of Robert McNamara, former US Defence Secretary, who was a dominating president from 1967 to 1981. McNamara was a man of ferocious will, personal commitment to alleviating poverty and frighteningly little common sense.*

A rigid belief that any investment leads to growth failed. The investments were unbalanced, with too much devoted to building roads and factories and not enough to health programs, for example. Another crucial problem was that the investments didn't hold the receivers accountable. No effective systems for oversight of the spending of the funds were put into place. Finally, the investments, because they were made in the form of loans, piled on debt, and the repayments required on those debts began to strangle economic growth in most of the developing countries. Ultimately, one country after another defaulted on the loans. Referring to this perverse outcome as he witnessed it unfold during his time at the World Bank, Martin Wolf wrote, "Every division found itself under great pressure to lend money, virtually regardless of the quality of projects on offer or of the development programmes of the countries. . . . [This] encouraged borrowers to pile up debt, no matter what the likely returns." His time at the bank was altogether "two wasted decades," Wolf said.

One telling example of the kind of misguided project that was so often funded is cited by William Easterly in his book *The Elusive Quest for Growth*, the case of Ghana's hydroelectric dam and aluminum plant. As Easterly told it, the project began in the 1950s with aid to dam the Volta River. They did that, creating the largest man-made lake in the world. The electricity from it would run an aluminum smelting plant, which would get aluminum from proposed mines in Ghana, thereby producing an aluminum industry. The new Lake Volta was also to provide a water transport route between north and south Ghana, and a large new fishing industry. But by the 1980s it was clearly a failure. The dam turned out electricity, but not profitably; aluminum was smelted, but the aluminum was imported, not mined in Ghana. The fisheries failed from poor administration and equipment. Eighty thousand people lost their homes in the creation of the lake, and then were driven away from the shores by an array of waterborne diseases, including river blindness, malaria, hookworm, and schistosomiasis. "The real disaster is that the Ghanaians are still about as poor as they were in the early 1950s," Easterly wrote. The project was attended by a fleet of troubles, including five coups in the country, but fundamentally there were simply no good guides about how to make such a thing work. Hundreds of such horribly failed projects could be described.

When a series of shocks to the global economy raised alarms in the 1990s, those economists who put forth analyses of the underlying problems in the world economic system turned their attention to the failure of the post–World War II efforts to spur development. Joseph Stiglitz, Jeffrey Sachs, William Easterly, and others took a hard look at the reasons for that failure, and what they found was that that there were three main factors that could help explain why development projects hadn't been more effective. First, aid had been far too strongly focused on infrastructure building instead of building human capital, including health and education. Second, aid programs were not designed to meet specific goals under the scrutiny of monitors, watching both for the results and for any possibility of misspending the money. Third, the projects were too small in dollars and ambition, as well as too brief.

The work of this rising generation of specialists has now been loosely synthesized into a new approach to development which has been given various names, but the most apt of which, I think, is "enlightened globalization." This approach, based on work across several fields, has brought to prominence the vital link between investment in public health and economic progress, a lesson learned way back in the mid-nineteenth century during England's battle against cholera.

Of course, England's investment in the battle against cholera was an investment at home, an easier case to make than that for spending public funds on projects in countries around the world. But then, with the increasing globalization of all facets of our lives, we can't afford to consider the problems in the developing world as not our own.

The new approach to aid is something different from what was delivered in the 1950s and 1960s. The work in the sciences and economics has given us new information. It has demonstrated that the investments in physical capital and top-down aid, basically, the Rostow approach that dominated ideas of aid in the past, was incomplete. What is required now is to fund on-the-ground projects developed from within the countries, like those profiled in the preceeding chapters. In what follows, the rationale for the new approach to aid will be explored. As policy analysts have said, such projects build not only health, but help build political stability and economic growth.

6

Investing in Health

A major moment in the rise to prominence of the enlightened globalism movement was the publication in 1993 of a bold report by the World Bank, in book form, titled, *Investing in Health*. It drew on several years' work by scholars who were just then rising to prominence; they are now stars in their own right: for example, Dean Jamison of UCLA, Christopher Murray and David Bloom of Harvard, Jeffrey Sachs of Columbia, and Richard Feachem of the Global Fund, among many others.

The bank had long been counted as among those pushing globalization forward too carelessly with a market fundamentalism that was dangerously rigid. But in publishing *Investing in Health*, the bank broke with decades of tradition.

The report suggested that the standard model of economics was missing something. It had pretty much started and ended with investment in physical capital. It was assumed that once some wealth was produced in a society health would follow later. In the 1993 report the bank suggested that investing in human capital—health and education—could be as powerful a lever as the traditional investments in roads, agriculture, and mining.

The report took health spending out of the category of charity and put it in the column of "most important investments." It put the case plainly: Much of human progress can be attributed to increases in wealth, but a large portion of our gains come because of health as well. It said, "Private markets will not give the poor adequate access" to health. Therefore, it is essential that governments do much more investing in health projects. Governments should spend less on ineffective health measures—such as big hospitals—"and instead double or triple spending on basic health programs such as immunizations and AIDS prevention and on essential clinical services." It suggested every country should finance a minimum package of services for all that would include prenatal and child care, family planning and treatment for such central diseases as AIDS, tuberculosis, and malaria. Economists and government leaders should not focus on growth alone, the report said, but must pay attention to equity and health as well.

Economists David Canning and David Bloom of Harvard explained the new approach to building wealth in poor countries in a 2004 article in *Science* magazine. They wrote:

> *a revolution in economic thinking has taken place over the last few decades, putting human capital, particularly educated workers, on a par with physical capital as an input in to production. We would argue . . . that increased health is another aspect of human*

capital that also enters into production. In addition, long life expectancy may be the fundamental force that creates the demand for education and encourages domestic saving that is a key determinant of growth. This perspective offers an exciting new possibility in international development: investing in health to help stimulate development.

The paper showed that health is more than just a factor in growth. Its effect "above and beyond other influences on economic growth, emerges consistently across studies, and is strikingly large." The authors give the example of two countries that are otherwise similar, but one has a life expectancy five years longer. Using real country data they found that the country with a somewhat longer life span will grow annually by 0.3 percent to 0.5 percent *more* every year than other nations. Given that the average growth among world nations between 1965 and 1990 was only 2 percent, this would be a very large figure. "Moreover," they wrote, "a gain of 5 years in life expectancy is well within the reach of most developing countries—since 1950, for example, life expectancy worldwide has increased by about 20 years."

The reason that health is such a fundamental driver includes several points that have so far been verified:

Productivity: Healthier people lose fewer days at work, and when they do go to work, they are more energetic and mentally alert. Illness in a household also often means that otherwise healthy people must cut work time to take care of someone else in the family who is ill.

Education: Healthier people who live longer have more incentive to increase their skills through education because they expect it will pay off. Healthier children and adults also attend school more regularly and drop out less often.

Investment in physical capital: People who live longer are pressed to save more for retirement. They will eventually have more access to capital and their incomes will rise. In addition, factors like savings and health are strong magnets for the foreign investment a nation needs.

Demographic dividend: This phrase refers to the observation that nations, as they develop, often change from having overall high death rates and large numbers of children per family to fewer deaths and fewer children per family, because they are confident the children will survive. This leads to a dividend in which healthy children become new workers and produce beyond the level of the previous generation.

This health dividend, they wrote, is the root cause of the "Asian Miracle." Several formerly poor and overpopulated countries began a great rise in economic growth in the second half of the twentieth century. These sudden rises came about "largely thanks to high rates of growth factor inputs—labor, physical capital, and human capital—rather than increase in total factor productivity. One reason for the increase . . . has been the effect of better health. Improvements in health, feasible at modest cost, preceded and helped catalyze the so-called miracle. Life expectancy increased from 39 years in 1960 to 67 years in 1990, with a concomitant decline in fertility."

One of the keys to the new analysis is the shift away from old ways of measuring progress in an economy. Just counting the Gross Domestic Product (GDP) per person will not tell whether only 1 percent of a population owns everything—the inequality in a society that is so important to stability. It will also not tell how many people in the society are sick, or how often. Now, economists are using new measures to try to include these vital factors to get a better picture of whether a nation is not only growing but growing in a healthy or a dangerous way.

One of the measures now used is "full income" instead of regular income. This adds dollar income to a figure for health—life expectancy. When used instead of just the GDP per person, it gives a startlingly different graphic picture of a nation's progress. The GDP alone dampens and obscures important trends. Bloom and Canning give the example of Kenya.

When AIDS was beginning to devastate Kenya in the 1980s and 1990s, economists had trouble finding the effects of the scourge in their figures. That was because there were using GDP per person. If "full income" is used, the charts appear quite different. Kenya's growth in the years from 1960 to 1980 as clearly more robust than GDP could show, and then when the AIDS crisis hit, "full income" measures showed the steep drop right away, even while GDP showed very small changes.

Another of the new measures being employed is called the DALY, pronounced "dally," the disability-adjusted life year, meaning the years of life lost plus the years of life marred by substantial disability. Years of life can tell economists about the extremes happening in society, life and death. But the DALY adds in a measure to count those between full health and death. It brings in sickness and disability as well. As Richard Feachem, one of the contributors to the report, explained, "The question became how can you buy the most dallies for your dollar?" Some interventions can buy a whole year of healthy life expectancy for $10 to $100. "That's a huge gain on your investment. But other interventions can cost $10 million to $100 million per DALY gained, such as end-stage care in big hospitals," he said.

After the World Bank report the next large step toward commitment to a new view of economics and development came when Gro Harlem Brundtland, head of the World Health Organization in the late 1990s, created the Commission on Macroeconomics and Health.

Brundtland brought in eighteen of the world's top economists and policy makers, including Sachs, Feachem, Fogel, Jamison, and Manmohan Singh, India's prime minister. The work was done by six teams under the leaders, and took two years, ending with a report that was clear and authoritative.

The economists named the central issues.

First, contrary to previous belief, struggling nations could become trapped in a development sink from which they could not climb out by themselves.

Second, it is the burden of disease that "stands as a stark barrier to economic growth, and therefore must be addressed frontally."

Third, it is relatively few diseases, and ones that could easily be treated or prevented, that were responsible for the greatest part of the poverty trap. It was clear that something could be done.

The nature of the problem had been mistaken for decades, the report said, and "this report offers a new strategy for investing in health." By delivering just the most cost-effective and simple interventions—such as vaccination and basic treatment of malaria, tuberculosis, and diarrhea—eight million to ten million lives could be saved each year in the poorest countries.

The lives and years of disability saved would amount to, by very conservative estimates, 330 million DALYs per year. In dollars, that would amount to about $200 billion to $500 billion saved annually. In addition, the change in health could accelerate growth in the poor nations and help to break the poverty trap by adding tens to hundreds of billions of dollars in growth.

Other studies made other, strong arguments why the rich countries should undertake a new aid regime—self-interest. The new studies illuminated the vital link between basic health care and the political stability of nations, and by extension of international politics. One of the most profound findings is that there is no better measure of a nation's stability than its rate of infant mortality.

That surprising result emerged from more than five years of work by university researchers in the United States, including Jack Goldstone and Ted Robert Gurr at the University of Maryland, Jennifer Brower and Peter Chalk at the Rand Corporation, and at the National Intelligence Council, led by John Gannon.

The researchers took advantage of the fact that in the past two decades huge amounts of information about human society had been amassed in computer databases. It had been collected because it is needed in narrow specialties—for example, travel figures in tourism. Each specialty had been pressed to know, using data, what is going on in the field. Led by Gurr, beginning in 1994, the idea was to use some of this great stream of data to look at the broader subject of "state failure." The failures include various kinds of catastrophes, including coups, ethnic wars, destructive revolutionary wars, genocides, and "adverse regime changes," among others. The object was to find things that failed states had in common so that trouble in a state could be forecast.

They began with more than thirteen hundred different variables and narrowed them down to the most important seventy-five or so, including such items as gross domestic product per person, population density, religious factors, civil rights indexes, and health statistics.

The researchers identified 135 state failures around the world between 1955 and 2001 in countries with populations greater than 500,000. They then tracked each of those countries through the years just before the failure, looking for the conditions present in failed states versus stable ones. They found a handful of crucial factors.

The key drivers of state failure they found were: low levels of quality of life as reflected, for example, in infant mortality statistics; regime type, with "partial democracy" being the most vulnerable to collapse; lack of openness to international trade and cooperation; and the presence of ethnic or religious conflict.

"The strongest influence on the risk of state failure," the report said, "was regime type. All other things being equal, we found the odds of failure to be *seven times* as high for partial democracies as they were for full democracies and autocracies." This was written before the war in Iraq (indeed, it might have been very difficult to publish it afterward).

Assuming that unstable regimes are widespread and a fairly obvious risk factor, the study then looked to the next most important factors and found that "quality of life" was the most important. They tried measuring it in a number of different ways, using combinations of wealth-and-health figures. But the best overall measure they found was a nation's rate of infant mortality.

The reason this turns out to be a sensitive measure of a nation's well-being is that it is linked to so many basics of life. The level of nutrition, of health services, of clean water and sewage, of education all directly affect the survival of children and the feeling of well-being in a family. Babies are the vulnerable ones, the ones whose sickness and death is the most common indicator of widespread problems.

The series of reports on state failure produced and updated in recent years provide the key links between health and politics. Not long after the state failure work began to produce results, scholars in universities, government, and think tanks began to take the next step—suggesting how policy should take advantage of the emerging knowledge. Because policy makers had never before included health matters, they began to refer to the news from scientists about emerging diseases and from scholars about state failure as "non-traditional threats."

The January 2000 National Intelligence Estimate, a report published annually by the CIA and the National Intelligence Council, was the first annual issue to emphasize health and poverty as key factors to be counted in thinking about foreign policy and national security. The report made clear that policy action should begin immediately because of the long time it would take to build up the systems that might catch epidemics early or avert health problems on the ground in poor countries. As noted earlier, the report said, "New and emerging infectious diseases will pose a rising global health threat, and will complicate U.S. and global security over the next 20 years. These diseases will endanger U.S. citizens at home and abroad . . . and exacerbate social and political instability in key countries and regions."

In 2003, researchers Brower and Chalk of the Rand Corporation spelled out the sea change taking place. They began with a wistful note: With the collapse of the Soviet Union and the Eastern bloc, it said, "It appeared that the world system could be on the threshold of an era of unprecedented peace and stability. Politicians, diplomats and academics alike began to forecast the imminent establishment of a new world order." This new order would be "managed by an integrated international system [and] based on the principles of liberal democracy and the free market." (I think it is not an accident that the sentiments and even the wording from 1914 is similar to lines like these written now.)

The Rand book authors wrote of the unease with which experts now face the world. In the new world order "turmoil and chaos are increasingly emanating from undefined sources, while violence itself is largely being used by the 'weak' not so much as a means of expressing identity but as a way of creating it."

What defines the current most important threats is their global character, their ability to reach across borders—disease, terrorism, environmental degradation. Direct military action has become increasingly off the point and more like a loose cannon on deck.

Brower and Chalk wrote that traditional notions of security based on nations and territories need to be revised. They suggested picking up another theory about security that was devised in the 1960s. The concept, created by psychologist W. E. Blatz, is called "human security," as opposed to "national security." The central idea is that the main focus of security should no longer be chiefly on nations but on individuals and their well-being. "It is an alternative way of seeing the world," said Canadian foreign minister Lloyd Axeworthy, "taking people as its point of reference, rather than focusing exclusively on the security of territory or governments."

This different viewpoint changes what's on the agenda. It moves to the most fundamental human issues first—health and wealth. Economist Ramesh Thakur described it this way: "Negatively, it refers to freedom from: want, hunger, attack, torture, imprisonment without a free and fair trial . . . and so on. Positively, it means freedom to: . . . [have] opportunities that allow each human being to enjoy life to the fullest. Putting the two together, human security refers to the quality of life of the people of a society."

Commentators recently have bickered about whether the United States is stingy or generous with aid, but that misses the point entirely. Steven Radelet, an economist with the Center for Global Development, wrote in *Foreign Policy* magazine that the key question is not whether we are doing a lot or a little, but "whether we are doing enough to achieve our own foreign policy goals in the developing world." He concluded, "Sadly, our efforts are woefully inadequate."

Colin Powell, after leaving his post in the Bush administration in 2005, wrote in *Foreign Policy* of today's issues:

None is more important than economic development in the world's poorest societies. . . . Development is not a "soft" policy issue, but a core national security issue. . . . We see a link between terrorism and poverty. Poverty breeds frustration and resentment, which ideological entrepreneurs can turn into support for—or acquiescence to—terrorism, particularly in those countries in which poverty is coupled with a lack of political rights and basic freedoms. . . . The United States cannot win the war on terrorism unless we confront the social and political roots of poverty.

Radelet in the same magazine added:

Unfortunately many citizens of poor countries see economic opportunity, escape from poverty and political freedom as distant dreams. The gap between the richest and poorest countries has widened considerably during the last 20 years, breeding bitterness and anger among people who believe—rightly or wrongly—that the rich have rigged the international system against them. A growing number of groups are promoting radical ideologies that see the United States as the problem, not the solution.

It is the growing momentum of the enlightened globalization movement, through such projects as the Millennium Development Project; the Global Fund to Fight AIDS, Tuberculosis and Malaria; and President Bush's Millennium Challenge Account, that if ramped up to new levels of funding, can begin to convince people from poor nations that they too can climb out of poverty. By providing adequate support for concerted funding of health projects of the type described earlier we will be committing to the most effective defense against the many threats confronting us in this challenging phase of globalization. Every dollar committed to such projects will be a powerful investment in the future health and stability of our world. That investment would change the tenor of politics in our era if the leading nations make good on their promises of aid for the new millennium.

7

If Not Now, When?

We have crossed a divide. It is no longer possible to go back to the comforting belief that that the developing world is hopeless and so we need do nothing. Some hope has developed, and even the beginning of expectations.

With the beginning of an enlightened globalism movement and several new international organizations to back it up, the attention turns to the leaders and the momentum that is building. Are they up to it, and will it take off?

One of those who is at the center of the activity is Richard G. A. Feachem, one of the contributors to the World Bank's 1993 *Investing in Health*. He is the director of the newly created Global Fund to Fight AIDS, Tuberculosis and Malaria. He's English, but with dark good looks that would not be out of place in any capital in the south ends of the planet.

His beard is fashionably short, peppered in black and gray, and he wears an international-gray suit. From his résumé, it is clear that

Feachem speaks four languages in addition to his own British English. But he rates himself truly fluent in only one other—Tok Pisin, one of the languages of Melanesia. Feachem also has degrees in engineering, medicine, and environmental health. The odd thing about this is that it is not rare anymore. Feachem is one of a growing cadre of double-cultured, multilingual leaders of development institutions.

On a mild winter's day in 2005 Feachem sits at a conference table in Washington, D.C., explaining the Global Fund. It is not only a new organization, but a new *type* of organization, he says. It is a stream-lined, fully independent financial NGO, the first of its kind.

Its job is to collect large-scale money from all kinds of donors— governments, companies, or citizens—and distribute it to health proj-ects in poorer nations. Its method is crucial and the reason for its existence. It is not a bureaucracy, not linked to governments or the United Nations. It gives grants, not loans, for projects created and proposed by groups in the countries themselves. The Global Fund vets the proposals, monitors spending, and measures how well the projects succeed in meeting their targets. The Global Fund is also committed to correcting the mistake of "vertical" rather than "hori-zontal" health programs; its funding gives half to infrastructure (such as computers, management training, nurses, and equipment) and half to direct medical needs like drugs and vaccines.

It is a rigorous system designed to avoid the problems that have plagued aid in the past four decades. Now the idea is to learn from ear-lier experience, to count and measure everything, to do and redo proj-ects until they work or are shut down. The Global Fund has the power to withdraw funds or stop projects at any moment if they are wasting money or not meeting their targets. It has so far collected and distributed about $3 billion, and hopes in the next few years to be receiving and giving about $8 billion per year.

There is no other organization that collects and distributes money in quite this way. For example, one of the early grants was given to the Ministry of Health in Ghana. But the Global Fund requires that the proposal come from a group that is broader than just government, so the fund helped Ghana set up a committee that includes citizens, businessmen, and nongovernmental organizations.

"This is new for us," says George Amofah, director of the public health division in Ghana's ministry of health. The "country coordinating mechanism," as it is called, "has brought in members of civil society as colleagues and friends. Together we develop proposals and work toward an agreed program of work. It's not easy. We have people with various levels of understanding of issues and differing agendas. To harmonize these interests one needs a lot of diplomatic tact and the ability to compromise."

The object is to challenge the local citizens to devise and control programs to meet their needs—"ownership" in the current jargon.

The goals are specific. For example, in Indonesia, one project is intended to treat fifty thousand tuberculosis patients with directly observed therapy (DOT), in which health care workers are present when patients take their medicine, to assure compliance. In the first year the goal was to treat 30,000 with the DOT method; the project actually included 39,000. But in another project, training laboratory technicians, the goal was 1,700 and only 1,555 were trained on time. Something will have to be done to make sure they don't slip farther behind, or the grant could be in trouble.

Rosmini Day, of the Indonesia department of health, says, "The point is that with the Global Fund, it is all time-bound. We are under pressure all the way through. Every three months we assess ourselves, and are assessed. No report, no money! It's a very direct kind of oversight; it is a quite new thing for us."

Despite such effective models for the distribution of aid, building support for large-scale increases in funding is still hobbled by the widespread perception that so much aid money has been wasted in the past. Feachem says that there are many myths about aid for health projects, and one of the most damaging is that huge sums of money have been spent on such projects in the past to little effect. In fact, the giving for health-specific projects has been tiny, and over the years has gotten even tinier.

"We were drip feeding," he says, "tiny, tiny increments of health funding. We were saying to developing countries things like, 'If you are spending $8 per person on health, we'll give you money to spend $8.50 per person and see what you can do with *that*.' This was just nonsense. The amounts of money needed to have an effect were much larger, especially for the hardest problems."

Aid for Africa in 2002, for example, amounted to a total of $30 per person from all the world's donors. And, as Jeffrey Sachs has written, of the $30 about $5 actually went to consultants from donor countries, $9 went to pay the countries' debts to Western countries, and $3 was for emergency food aid. That left only $12 that actually went as aid to

Africa. From the United States in the same year, after deductions like those above, about 6 *cents* per person was given. It would be astonishing if any concrete results had come out of such small sums.

The effort has simply not been a serious attempt to get results. At the start of the Marshall Plan the United States gave almost 3 percent of its GDP to foreign aid. That figure has dropped steadily year by year, to the point that the United States now gives about 0.16 percent of GDP—about one-nineteenth of the earlier rate.

Unfortunately, the myth of high spending is alive and well, as polls over the years have shown. When Americans were asked how much their country is spending on foreign aid, they guessed a figure that was about twenty-five times higher than the United States actually spends. When told the true figure most Americans agree that the country spends too little, and they would be willing to put in more. (The money is *so* small: Just what is lost each year to tax cheats in the United States is twenty times more.)

Another of the myths about aid is that corruption is the reason why aid goes astray and is ineffective. But there are criteria that international groups such as the World Bank, Transparency International, and Freedom House use to measure corruption, and the pattern in these measures does not fit the mythology. What they show is that very poor countries around the world have higher corruption scores, and their scores improve as they become more prosperous. The rankings show that African countries are not on average more corrupt than, say, countries in Asia. More important, it is clear from cases like Bangladesh that aid and development can be very successful even while the government is corrupt. It is just necessary to deliver aid through other organizations; in fact, delivered that way, the government ministers can see effective programs and learn from them.

Momentum has, nonetheless, been building for substantial increases in funding for the new generation of aid programs, and it has been fueled by both realistic assessments of the specific amount of money required and a growing consensus among prominent analysts and world leaders.

One source of solid—and compelling—numbers for the amount of new aid required is the report issued in 2001 by the World Health Organization's Commission on Macroeconomics and Health. At the time the report was written the world was spending about $6 billion on development aid. The commission said the number would have to increase to about $27 billion to cover the basics.

A package of essential services could be had for about $34 per person in poorer nations, the commission calculated. (For comparison, the United States spent $4,500 per person annually. Only Americans paid that much for health care; other leading nations paid about $2,500 at the time, still a long way above the needed $34.) The commission figured that the poor countries themselves could come up with the first $15 needed, and donors could supply the other $19 per year. For the wealthy countries it would amount to an increase in spending of about 0.1 percent of their GDPs.

Another hopeful discovery revealed in the report is that the great burden of disease in poor countries results from just a few conditions and that they are the ones that are treatable with relatively cheap means.

The commission calculated what was needed was fifty billion dollars a year above current commitments, but it cautioned that

these financial targets are a vision of what should be done, rather than a prediction for what will happen. We are all too aware of donor countries that neglect their international obligations despite vast wealth, and of recipient countries that abjure the governance needed to save their own people. Maybe little increased funding will take place; donors might give millions when billions are needed and impoverished countries will fight wars against people rather than disease, making it impossible for the world community to help. We are not naïve: it is no accident that millions of people— voiceless, powerless, unnoticed by the media—die unnecessarily every year.

Nations had already agreed more than once to begin raising the level of aid by a large amount, but the promises remained unfulfilled.

The commission's report offered a powerful summary statement about why it is crucial that this time around the developed nations follow through.

With globalization on trial as never before, the world must succeed in achieving its solemn commitments to reduce poverty and improve health. The resources—human, scientific, and financial— exist to succeed, but now must be mobilized. As the world embarks on a heightened struggle against the evils of terrorism, it is all the

more important that the world simultaneously commit itself to sus-
taining millions of lives through peaceful means as well, using the
best of our modern science and technology and the enormous wealth
of the rich countries. This would be an effort that would inspire and
unite peoples all over the world.

We've seen hopeful signs that serious commitments will be made. On a sunny morning in May 2001, in the Rose Garden at the back of the White House, President Bush announced that the United States would make the founding contribution to the Global Fund to Fight Aids, Tuberculosis and Malaria, $200 million at the time, with more to follow. On either side of him that day were UN Secretary-General Kofi Annan and Nigerian president Olusegun Obasanjo. Annan spoke to reporters, saying the beginning of the Global Fund to Fight AIDS, Tuberculosis and Malaria was a crucial step. "I believe today will be remembered as the day we turned the tide," Mr. Annan said.

An array of leaders with different views and styles pressed the matter of aid forward. Japan had been the first to propose a global fund, and Jacques Chirac of France strongly supported it. After George Bush committed $200 million, the European Union committed $300 million more to get the fund started. Tony Blair of England pledged new levels of aid and called for $25 billion in new aid to Africa alone.

Support for health funding has even begun to develop among conservatives and religious figures in America and Britain. Davis Bunn, a best-selling author of Christian novels, has become a member of the board of the Global Fund to Fight AIDS, Tuberculosis and Malaria. It seems somehow a natural update to the missionary tradition in Christianity.

Richard Horton, the cautious editor of *The Lancet,* said he thought maybe a fundamental gulf had been bridged. People had dropped the old view of "Africa as an impossible continent, full of corruption and conflict."

"Three important areas of broad consensus have emerged," he wrote. First, the mission has been agreed on around the world, as nations signed on to the Millennium Development Goals. Second, the political framework for achieving the goals is agreed to be strengthening of democracies. And third, the economic case for the critical part that health plays in development has been largely accepted.

With international momentum slowed by the distractions of war, the next steps have become more difficult—but more necessary at the same time. Five steps are needed now to move ahead. First, the major countries must commit to large increases in aid, and a timetable for the payments announced. Second, reform of the IMF and the World Bank must be undertaken to make them more transparent and to give smaller countries a voice in their policies. Third, the Global Fund to Fight AIDS, Tuberculosis and Malaria or a successor should be put forward as the chief financing mechanism of much of the new aid. Fourth, an international research and consulting agency must be created to carry on the study of the most important diseases and how to combat them. Fifth, a large public information campaign to lay out the issues and name the choices should be undertaken immediately.

What has developed is a mode in which we are now moving along two paths simultaneously—one that will assure failure and one that may make it work. It is not a race to the bottom or the top. Right now, it is both.

Now we are combating terrorism, fending off protests, watching as more nations than ever fail, and trying to shore up the international system while it shambles toward a moment when a single spark will set it alight again. The one thing that is clear is that something substantial has been missing from the international system. It is out of balance. If we just start from Adam Smith's outline and use a bit of hindsight, it's not hard to see what's missing.

Smith said markets were inherently inadequate by themselves. The systems must be governed, and while the private goods flow, governments must provide some public goods that cannot be supplied by the market and its self-interested action. He suggested ways to draw off a portion of the great stream to maintain the system. Over the years, nations have decided how much they should invest in their schools, roads, fire, police, health, and environmental works. In the United States the amount is about $30 of every $100. Despite arguments about it, that number has not changed greatly in many decades.

But turning to the international system, the amount of the world flow put in to uphold it has been fatally small. The industrial nations together spend not 10 percent of their production, or 1 percent, but closer to 0.25 percent.

It is reasonable that the global figure should be lower than national spending on public goods because the nations and businesses themselves provide much infrastructure that is needed. On the other hand, world trade and international communication create needs that do not exist for nations separately.

The figure expressing what is needed by the international system has been calculated a number of times, and a base figure has been agreed on in principle by nations for more than thirty years. It is about 0.7 percent of the GDP of the industrial nations—$0.70 for every $100 of production. The United States now spends about $13 of every $100 on personal health, more than $20 on defense, and $20 on social security, but only $0.16 on aid. This is the nation's fundamental investment in making the international system work.

As Bob Geldof said, "We say we are a free-trade society. Adam Smith is clear in *The Wealth of Nations*; he says infant societies must be protected. You are a free trader; read the Bible!"

There is now an historic chance to adjust the international system to what we know are good principles. From our experience before the first two great wars we already know what happens when leading groups in society take out much and put back little. There is first resentment, then anger and protest, and then violence. More important than each of these is that the heart of the whole system is threatened. The system itself is slouching toward illegitimacy in the eyes of many; when that moment is reached, collapse can be triggered by seemingly small and even apparently unrelated events.

We have significant advantages over earlier attempts to make a world system work. We now have reasonable calculations of how much money is needed. We now have a better idea of how important monitoring and accountability are. We know that some goals must be explicit and that they take continuous work to reach and maintain. We now know something even more vital—where to put the money. We must start now with human capital, well-monitored.

This is a general plan and not a panacea. But it is an exhilarating plan. To Adam Smith, holding in his hands our knowledge would have seemed a great gift from God and a sin if we did not use them.

We have built up a platform to a great height, but what we are doing now is halting before building the supports and allowing rust and wind to test it constantly. What we don't know is how long we have before our mistakes overtake our successes. But if we fail, it will be a long fall and a hard landing.

Is a rescue plan like that offered by Sachs realistic? Definitely not, unless you count the Marshall Plan or the eradication of smallpox as "realistic." They weren't, but that of course is what makes humans human. Things can get done when people begin to believe.

When Jeffrey Sachs published *The End of Poverty*, a book that contains a bold plan to try to eliminate not all poverty, but the worst of it around the world, the reviews were consistent. Yes, it's a noble and worthy goal, but it's unlikely to happen. From *The New York Times:* "It's highly unlikely that Sachs's proposals will ever be adopted in full." From *The New Yorker:* "Aid is not a panacea, and, even if the funding Sachs wants were to materialize, his grandest objectives may well remain unfulfilled."

Yet, from behind the casual journalistic cynicism, there was clearly some yearning for a different way. The *Times* reviewer, a conservative political science professor at the University of Chicago, wrote, "Even if 'The End of Poverty' is only half right, the payoff would be enormous: more than 500 million people helped. Sachs hasn't found a sure thing. But that doesn't mean his bet should not be made."

The New Yorker reviewer, economics writer John Cassidy, said,

"Here's another way to look at it: to pay for the extra spending, each American would have to contribute less than the cost of buying a cappuccino from Starbucks once a week. But, targeted carefully, aid can reward responsible governments, encourage individual initiative, and alleviate suffering. Surely that's worth a cup of coffee."

The war in Iraq and the rising tides of anti-Americanism could derail enlightened globalization, or any globalization. But that is exactly the reason why a grand plan to attack disease and poverty in the poorest countries can work. It would be unexpected, especially if led by the United States, and it would refresh the world memory about what they liked about America in earlier eras.

The reserve of goodwill is clearly present; it needs only to be tapped by leadership.

When the Marshall Plan was proposed it was met with precisely the same kind of cynicism and skepticism. The warnings at the time were that the communists would derail international cooperation and would certainly sink the Marshall Plan. But the leadership in America put together a campaign to build a movement for it (intentionally, to avoid partisanship, it was not closely identified with Truman's White House, but much of the credit indeed goes to Truman).

So it was the creation of the "dubious" and "unlikely" Marshall Plan in 1947 that started the second globalization. It was a sort of clever form of charity.

Generosity has always been a bit suspect in our culture. But it can have its uses. In the time of Edwin Chadwick, the push to take care of workers' health was seen as liberal "weakness." The "strong" attitude was that people should take care of their own problems and pull themselves up without help. This theme of what is weak and what is strong recurs in politics often. But we have the advantage of looking back. We can see now that the workers of the time were not weak and they were not lazy. Cleaning up filth and disease was not "coddling weakness." It was a simple and practical step, a rational choice. In that time, strength was in seeing things as they were and making the rational choice in the face of passionate self-interest.

We have found through bloody experience and a few revolutions that there are limits to how much unfairness will be tolerated. Beneath the choice to provide clean water for all was the simple assertion that, while we expect inequality and tolerate some injustice because we don't know an easy way to improve the system, there are some inequalities that are both wrong and destructive. If the rules are too unfair, it will not only hobble some runners in a race, but will eventually wreck the race itself. It will destroy the legitimacy of the contest.

Was the building of sewers a needless public expense? Did it send the wrong message, to have the general public rather than the workers themselves pay for sewers? Was it charity or an essential service for a successful society? I put the question that way because charity is often counted as a kind of softness, merely an effort to relieve suffering; nice, but not required. It is not thought of as very important in the framework of society, and it is even said to be dangerous if it becomes coddling and creates dependency in those who receive it. Thus, in Chadwick's day, the reformers spent a lot of energy trying to deny that their projects were charity. Providing sewers—formerly purchased only by those who could afford them—was really necessary, and in the self-interest of the whole society. It was necessary to maintain the legitimacy of government's contract with the people. At the time, a huge antigovernment movement was rising, riots were occurring with regularity, and the signs of health in society were sinking. The choice in hindsight was sensible enough. The facts have demonstrated that the reformers were right—sanitation is practical and bankable.

There is a story nearer our own time that is similar, an even better lesson in what is strength and what is weakness. It is a lesson we can use now.

The story of the Marshall Plan pivots on one day, a Tuesday, April 29, 1947. On that day General George Catlett Marshall, the U.S. secretary of state, was upset; and he was beginning to see the state of the world much differently than he had before. He was about to take action.

Marshall was a soldier's soldier, a man of few, blunt words. He was what used to be called a "slow learner" in school, like Einstein, but he had an unusual power to see events in perspective. He was one of the greatest heroes of that time, and Churchill gave him credit for being the "true organizer of the victory" in World War II.

President Harry Truman had some limitations as a leader, but he had one excellent combination of talents—he could understand how people saw him, including the unflattering bits. In addition, he was a good judge of talent. So, after the war, when the peace was going badly and Europe was injured and ailing, in danger of becoming a permanent invalid, Truman called General Marshall out of retirement to become secretary of state. He had won the war and the respect of everyone; now Marshall would have to win the peace.

In his new job, the crucial test came as he set off for Moscow in March 1947. Even two years after the war there was no treaty and no decisions about what to do with renegade Germany and Austria. The jockeying among nations for position in the coming world was still underway. Marshall left on March 5 and visited Europe on his way to the showdown in Moscow.

He knew Europe from his war years in the fields of France. Marshall's career had started before the first world war; he had gone to the front as a staff officer in charge of planning. He had witnessed the first mass loss of life in Saint-Mihiel and in Argonne Forest in France in 1917 and 1918, experiences that had changed him deeply.

Now he was back, after a second great war over the same turf. There had been drought in Europe; bread lines were everywhere. Industry had never been rebuilt after the war, and a total collapse seemed at hand. Europe looked like it might become one of those places that were perpetually poor and without prospect of recovery. It had happened to other great regions in many eras, in just this way. French farmers could not get supplies to sow their fields, so they grew what they could, not for the market, but just to feed their animals and themselves. German workers were getting only half of what they needed in their diets to do a day's work. Food aid was needed for hundreds of thousands, just to avoid starvation. The coldest winter in decades was coming, and that would divert fuel to home heating, with little left over to supply business and industry. The roads, railroads, houses, and fields that had been destroyed in the war were not yet rebuilt, even two years later.

"What is Europe now?" asked Winston Churchill. "It is a rubble heap, a charnel house, a breeding ground of pestilence and hate." Would there be riots, angry political movements running across the continent? There was a struggle for power among the surviving nations, and rumors of coups. This meant to Marshall that, beyond all reason, the world was headed in precisely the disastrous direction it had gone after World War I. There would be more bickering, instability, and worse, possibly even another general war. At that moment the governments of Eastern Europe were already shaky.

The conference in Moscow was intended to lay down the basic outlines of a treaty on Germany and Austria. Marshall thought there were grounds for negotiation. He had worked well with the Soviets on the field during the war, and assumed they would approach the peace in a similar, practical way. He felt both the United States and the Soviet Union would be seeking some stability, some rules under which both nations could rebuild and go forward. Each side in the war now occupied a number of countries. How would they, most importantly Germany, be governed? Under what rules would former Nazi states be allowed to conduct commerce, government, and defense?

But after he arrived in Moscow, Marshall was forced to sit through day after day of frustrating discussions with Foreign Minister Vyacheslav Molotov; no common ground appeared, only a swamp of rhetoric. Marshall wondered if it was just Molotov who was completely intransigent, so he went to meet with Stalin himself. But that meeting was even worse. Stalin doodled sketches of a wolf's head as Marshall spoke; Stalin's final position was to say that it really made no difference whether agreement was reached about Europe now. When the starvation of Germans and others was raised, he said that Russia had suffered so much from Germany, feelings of compassion toward Germans were inconceivable.

Marshall was shocked. Gradually, he realized that Stalin and the Soviet Union had no interest in pulling Europe out of trouble, or in rebuilding what had been there before. He realized then that the Soviets had a different agenda entirely, one which depended not on peace, but on turmoil. "It was my feeling," he wrote later, "that the Soviets were doing everything possible to achieve a complete breakdown of Europe. That is, they were doing anything they could think of to create greater turbulence."

As Marshall returned disheartened from Moscow, he got new intelligence reports saying that the United States had "grossly underestimated" the destruction in Europe and the ability of its people to come back.

So it was on that Tuesday after Marshall returned from Moscow that he instructed his key policy man, George Kennan, "to assemble a special staff 'immediately' and to report 'without delay' on what should be done to save Europe," as historian David McCullough has recalled.

Another war, Marshall felt, was the wrong answer. Marshall had to build stability in Europe even as Russia was trying to undermine it. There needed to be a different way forward. The great war was over, but still there was no peace. America had already given hundreds of millions of dollars in aid to unstable countries in Europe, yet they were shakier than ever. What could possibly be the way forward?

The climate was not good for dramatic plans, so at first he worked quietly. In America there were calls for punitive measures against Germany—asking for $10 billion in reparations and forcing Germany to cede control of its coal regions and industrial area to outsiders.

"A rebellious House of Representatives," as Marshall biographer Ed Cray wrote, "at that moment was hacking a $350 million foreign aid bill down to $200 million; State Department protests that the cut meant starvation and despair for 35 million people in Europe had been disregarded." Greece and Turkey were in danger of collapsing and even falling to communist coups, but the House had halted bills that would spend money to support them.

Marshall and his staff, working with the White House, created a plan that was bold and essentially outside all government experience. It was about aid, but it was not charity. It was something qualitatively different, both on an entirely new scale and using different rules. The plan contemplated not one year of aid, but sustained aid for four years—at least. The money requested would not be millions, but *billions*—a total of $17 billion (more than $200 billion in today's dollars). That was the largest project of its kind ever proposed.

Also, it would not follow the usual pattern of emergency aid. It would not be money sent like a telegram from the donor. Rather, it required the countries asking for it to analyze their own needs, and to draw up practical plans for achieving them. Then, only then, the

United States would fund the worthy plans. The object was to get something concrete done, not as in the past, simply to make vaguely helpful gestures.

Among the most important provisions was that the aid would come in the form of grants, not loans. During the period after World War I many private speculators gave loans to strapped nations and interests, but those added a burden of debt in an already bad situation, created resentment of the system that produced the indebtedness, and lost the speculators a lot of money in the process.

Allen Dulles, writing about the different approach of the Marshall Plan, said, "The United States has given all the old-style help it can. The United States has lent or given money and goods to individual countries without any overall plan. It is useless to do this any longer."

Further, the plan *included enemies*—an approach described as the first of its kind by any victorious nation. The plan included not only Germany but also the newly hostile Soviet Union and other communist countries.

All this was startling. The first time the financial numbers reached the Senate Foreign Relations Committee, committee leaders assumed they were simply mistakes; they were astronomically high. Then, the notion that our most hated enemy of two years before would now get money from us, and that our likely enemy of the future could also benefit, was met with astonishment. (As, perhaps, large amounts of health aid sent to Muslim countries today would be.)

That, said former West German chancellor Willy Brandt, was the genius of it. It put the aid morally above all contention. It was true humanitarian work. It also cleverly assumed that the best organized and best intentioned countries—ourselves of course included—were likely to benefit the most.

Selling the plan would not be easy. The initial polls showed that most Americans knew nothing of it, or opposed it. It was "hopeless," opponents said. It would be just throwing good money after bad. Foreign aid was counted as a waste of money. The phrase "pouring money down a rat hole" was used (and still echoes from the Senate in our time). Senator Arthur Vandenberg, chairman of the Senate Foreign Relations Committee, objected to the idea of "opening the treasury to every country in the world."

Marshall built a movement to push the plan forward. It included the 1940s equivalent of a TV campaign—that is, speeches on radio and talks at meetings and events all over the country by a variety of speakers. There were articles and books.

Marshall himself was the first to present it publicly, at the 1947 graduation ceremony at Harvard University. The plan didn't have a name, but wily Harry Truman called it the "Marshall Plan." Marshall objected, but Truman said Marshall had better follow the orders of the commander-in-chief. With Marshall's name on it, it had a chance; with Truman's it would be torn to shreds.

The chief selling point was made by Marshall at the beginning of the campaign, and consistently throughout: This is not charity. We are only helping the Europeans to help themselves, and we will benefit besides.

The plan spoke directly to the problem of a deeply interconnected world, a problem that the nations had failed to address after World War I. Marshall said that "countries must be self-supporting for there to be stability and peace . . . [and without help] recovery would take so long as to give rise to hopelessness despair and fear." He added, "Hopeless people often resort to desperate measures."

Americans must "face up to the vast responsibility which history has clearly placed upon our shoulders. . . . The whole world's future hangs on proper judgment, hangs on the realization of the American people of what can be done, of what must be done."

And, said Allen Dulles, "it is not a philanthropic enterprise." Americans of course were always generous in giving relief—during the Russian crop failure and starvation in 1921, during the earthquake in Japan in 1923. But the Marshall Plan, he said, is not that kind of undertaking. "It is an integral part of American policy. It is based on our views of the requirements of American security, . . . the only peaceful avenue now open to us which may answer the communist challenge to our way of life and our national security."

Undersecretary of State William Clayton, a Texas millionaire and an isolationist before the war, pitched it this way: "Let us admit right off that our objective has as its background the needs and interests of the people of the United States. We need markets—big markets—in which to buy and sell."

Kiplinger magazine, one of the most popular business magazines of the time, produced a special issue on the Marshall Plan, and put the matter in classical 1950s ad language: "The Marshall Plan is very much a business plan. . . . At its root is an office and factory and warehouse job. The Marshall Plan means work, and you will be one of the workers. . . . Now you've got it . . . what are you going to do about it? Do you think it's a matter for diplomats? The ideology is a thing of the past. Now the plan is down to earth, smack on your desk, a shirt-sleeves job. You will make the stuff, sell the stuff, ship the stuff."

Allen Dulles went one step beyond the business argument. "Critics say dollars will not save Europe. There is an element of truth in that. . . . Weapons alone will not do it either." There is a need for a spiritual force, "a force that will grip men's minds," as he put it. It was the force of hope, of people building up their families and their countries.

"It is only by restoring the economic life of a country . . . that we can meet the threat of dictatorship," Dulles said. We would thus confront extremism "not with arms or atomic bombs, but with a restored economic life for the men and women of Western Europe."

What got the Marshall Plan passed in Congress, finally, was not just the campaign on its behalf. It was the communist coup in Czecho-slovakia and the dramatic story during the coup that moderate foreign minister Jan Masaryk was thrown from his office window to his death. The alarm over Czechoslovakia made the Marshall Plan appear a brilliant antiterrorist piece of legislation. It was, British foreign minister Ernest Bevin said, "a turning point in world history," a credible, peaceful way to build democracy and capitalism and to seize the advantage from revolutionaries.

The period of the Marshall Plan came to be called the beginning of the European renaissance. The years 1948 to 1952 marked the fastest growth period in European history; industrial production rose 35 percent. Some of that boom must have come from the efforts and aid of the previous three years, but the new, targeted money added much fuel. Some historians have said the Marshall Plan's greatest worth was in the hope it gave Europe and the rules that were set down for the cooperative international economy of the coming decades.

There is, in that moment, some food for thought about our own times. Some of the problems seem rooted in the same basic issues we face now. We now also have many nations that are unstable: As noted earlier, there have been more breakdowns and more wars in the past twenty years than in previous decades. There are now also forces which gain not from peace and cooperation but from disruption, because they have a new ideological agenda for the world. We also have gone to war, and now are facing the prospect of a very difficult peace.

Could we generate the political will for such a plan now, a Marshall Plan–style program with developing countries as the beneficiaries?

Stories about the Marshall Plan have become stock images in the rhetoric of foreign policy. President Bush himself spoke of rebuilding Afghanistan in the way "America fed and rebuilt Japan and Germany." Skeptics quickly pulled out their history texts; *The New Yorker* magazine even before the end of 2001 carried an article on the "Marshall Plan Myth."

Politicians, the article said, "love to invoke the Marshall Plan as an example of how countries destroyed by war can be rebuilt almost overnight. In the popular imagination, the Marshall Plan transformed the economies of Europe, in just a few years, from ruined shells into vibrant industrial powerhouses. . . . But the Marshall Plan wasn't what we think it was."

Europe didn't go from zero to sixty in just the four years of the plan, 1948–1952. Substantial aid had already been provided. Walt W. Rostow, the giant figure of American development economics between the 1960s and 1980s, himself wrote after the collapse of the Soviet Union that the success of the Marshall Plan may have "generated the false hope that the application of capital and technology could do for Third World countries . . . what was achieved in Western Europe in the wake of World War II. Unlike these areas, Western Europe did not need to be invented; it simply had to be recalled."

What is interesting is that the Marshall Plan has again been invoked and argued over as we head into the new century. That is precisely because of its mythical power. It laid out a nonmilitary alternative. It was a program that is recalled not only in the United States, but all over the world, because it was admired for its spirit. It looked like real, practical leadership. While the United States did have a strong hand in guiding the plan and making sure the money was spent well, the plans were drawn up by Europeans. It is really not so much the details of the old plan that are now being invoked, it is the general approach.

Some of the specifics are still good places to start, but the circumstances of history are different. The original Marshall Plan would not work in Tanzania or Nepal. Rostow wrote (in 1997) that in thinking about the Marshall Plan in the twenty-first century, two things should be borne in mind—it was built in the United States in a bipartisan fashion, and it worked multi-laterally. "It provided the essential element of dignity and partnership to even the smallest partners. In the 21st century, the diffusion of power makes it even more essential that plans of action be arrived at on a multi-lateral basis."

Much has been done since 1948, even outside of Europe. The world is far richer; the pool of the poor is relatively smaller. And no one is asking to build "industrial powerhouses" in small nations; what is looked for is some provably worthwhile aid and an infusion of hope. There is no suggestion that all the poorest countries be included, or that grants be made in the face of corruption and inefficiency in some countries. William Easterly, former World Bank economist and no fan of foreign aid, suggested competitive grants might work better, and the incentives must be built in not only for nations, but for the people in the nations whom we want to succeed.

Probably the most encouraging and compelling reason to believe that a big new push of health aid today would produce striking results is the host of innovative, highly cost-effective programs working today on the ground developed by visionary people working within their home countries. Many of these projects, such as those visited earlier in the book, have been remarkably simple in conception, but with large payoffs.

These successes must drive us to support the push to fully fund this new breed of projects. Winston Churchill, stated the situation precisely as well as poetically, when facing the proposed rebuilding of Europe in 1948. He said that if at such a time we allow ourselves to be rent by pettiness and small disputes, if we fail in clarity of view or courage in action, a priceless occasion may be cast away forever. But if we all pull together and firmly grasp the larger hopes of humanity. Then it may be that we will move into "a happier sunlit age when all the children who are now growing up in this tormented world may find themselves not the victors nor the vanquished in the fleeting triumphs of one country over another, but the heirs of all the treasures of the past and the masters of all the science, the abundance, the glories of the future."

Conclusion

The Tale of Glass on the Beach:
Is It Prudent to Hope?

The project to enlist grandmothers in Nepal, the house-to-house polio campaign in India, the fight against killer diarrhea in the villages of Bangladesh, and giving the hope of new life to those infected with HIV in Botswana, have all been important because they have been successful or pointed the way, and there are many more such projects that have been proven on the ground. That point was brought home as I was writing this book, when a research volume appeared, called *Millions Saved: Proven Successes in Global Health*. It documents seventeen cases of successful projects. By coincidence, the seventeen were not the ones I happened to choose; none of the cases I describe here is included in that book, which suggests that successful and interesting cases are numerous.

The fact that such a book could be produced is a landmark in itself; the approach, the methods and measurements, the cases themselves are relatively recent but are compelling.

The book was the result of a research project led by Ruth Levine, director of research projects at the Center for Global Development, a nonprofit group in Washington, D.C., and a program of the center, called the What Works Working Group. It is another of the growing body of organizations pressing for more international health aid and a new way of thinking by national governments about how their foreign policy can shape the world.

The group, with help from the Centers for Disease Control and the National Institutes of Health in the United States, brought together fifteen experts in international health and economics and asked them to find and evaluate large-scale successes among health projects.

The group selected cases that shared five important features: They were all large, on a national to global scale; they addressed major public health problems; they showed a clear and measurable impact (not on secondary measures such as whether more children were immunized, but on the all-important direct measures: Only genuine changes in sickness and death were counted); they all worked over periods of at least five years; they were all highly cost-effective, one hundred dollars or less spent for each DALY (disability-adjusted life years; years of life gained, plus disability-free years gained).

Finally, the project took the logical step of abstracting from successful cases the lessons needed to create more successes. They are much like the ones pointed out here; the researchers enumerated six general findings about the successes. Several of them are counterintuitive, or offer evidence to correct myths about aid projects.

First, success is possible even in the poorest of countries. The hardest-to-reach poor can be found and helped significantly, even where governments are dysfunctional or corrupt; well-run programs can avoid running afoul of these traditional hazards.

Second, governments in poor countries may not have much money, but they can put some of their money and other resources into projects. They can carry out a substantial amount of the work needed for them. In most successful cases the governments not only helped, but were integral to the project's success.

Third, technology such as drugs and new computer and communication advances are eye-catching elements of success, but some of the best programs are built around behavior change, low-tech solutions, and house-to-house footwork.

Fourth, international coalitions have worked. The relatively new "public-private partnerships," of which there are now more than a dozen significant projects, offer another approach that does not depend wholly on the usual players—the wealthy donor nations, the United Nations, and the World Bank. Rather, private companies, NGOs, and the governments of poor nations can collaborate on large projects on their own.

Fifth, though in the past aid programs were not able to connect their efforts directly to gains in health, it is now possible. The working group found that proof of direct effects could be found, and should now be a routine part of evaluating projects.

Sixth, programs of many different types can work, from highly vertical ones that bring in something from the outside such as drugs or vaccines, along with outside experts to help organize the project, to highly horizontal ones that rely on local experts and local residents to work in villages; after accepting some outside help, they take over the work as their own. Most programs these days offer some combination of down-from-above help and local ownership.

"Major public health efforts can and have changed the world for the better—well beyond what would have occurred through income growth alone," the book noted. The proved cases in the book "put to rest the notion that nothing works in global health. But it raises new challenges: the first is how we make sure there are more and even bigger successes in the future."

We have both the know-how and the financial means to extend progress to the poorest people in the poorest places. We have never been as well equipped intellectually, financially, or technically to raise the level of health and wealth of society globally.

We must remember how far we've come, and that a good deal more is still possible, a point driven home to me one warm evening in October 1987, in Naples, not long after AIDS had first revealed itself to humanity. Beside the Castel dell'Ovo that reaches out over the water into the Bay of Naples Jonathan Max Mann walked on the cobbles next to the ancient stone walls. The evening had a sense of depth to it; here the Roman Empire came to its symbolic end, and the last emperor was imprisoned inside these walls in the fifth century.

The meeting that night was only the second time Western and African doctors were meeting to discuss the new epidemic. Dr. Mann, mustached and wearing his trademark bow tie, was chief of the Global Program on AIDS of the WHO. An American doctor from Boston, he first had had his mettle tested in the Congo—in the streets of Kinshasa and in the bush that stretches east for a thousand miles.

That night, as a reporter about to embark on a journey to the worst places of the epidemic in Africa, I wondered if Jon Mann was discouraged. He was leading an ill-supported fight against a foe that could not even be named in many places. The world was on the brink of what seemed then the strangest thing: a new infectious disease after we thought we had conquered infectious disease. Civilization on that evening seemed a boat riding on the moving magma of hot biology.

The new plague was beginning to be compared to the greatest diseases of human history—the Black Death, which killed a third of Europe's entire population, and the great influenza, which in a single year, 1918, killed some 40 million people, the worst carnage ever produced in a short time by any disease. The new HIV disease was on an epidemic rampage. It was not clear where new epicenters might open, or when.

I took Dr. Mann aside. Before asking for quotations for the record, I asked him as a person about what he felt. There were points of light on the black bay water when he looked at me kindly and gave me a lesson in public health history. Yes, AIDS was bad. It was worse to realize that it was not just the virus that was killing us, but our own behavior toward each other. This virus was just the latest thread of biological material that was able to employ our social inequities against us.

It *was* very discouraging. Then, he added, Speaking of great and continuing poverty and inequity did not carry us very far. "After you have said poverty is at fault, then what?" he asked. It's necessary to generate enough hope to do one or two useful things, he said. And charity isn't enough. Giving alone doesn't suggest a place to grasp, if the idea is to climb up from where we are. It's important to keep before us a few handholds to reach for so that we can continue upward, instead of just sticking fast and hoping things won't deteriorate.

As we walked back toward the noise and lights of Naples, he said it was always vital to remember that we had just come through a period in human history in which more people were healthier and productive than at any time since the dawn of the species. Few had ever been hopeful along the way, but much had been done anyway.

The job really was not to move the entire species from a dead stop but to lend a shoulder to keep the already generated momentum going.

"Easier," he said, smiling. "Much easier, no?"

That final point came home to me years later, about what progress had already been achieved and how we needed to keep going. I was reading an essay by Stephen Jay Gould. Things in the world are, of course, unjust, inhumane, and very hard to change. But, as Gould says, "I can hardly think of a more common, or sillier, fallacy of human thought and feeling than our propensity to construct 'golden age' myths about a simpler past of rustic bliss. . . . If anyone tells me he would rather have lived a century ago, I will simply remind him of the one irrefutable trump card for choosing right now as the best world we have ever known: thanks to modern medicine, people of adequate means in the industrial world will probably enjoy a privilege never before vouchsafed to any human group. Our children will grow up; we will not lose half or more of our offspring in infancy or childhood." We will not have to sing the "Songs on the Death of Children" or hire the daguerreotypist to take the only image of a dead child as it lay before the funeral.

Gould wrote that the deaths of children were among the most important events in the lives of both of the greatest heroes of his own profession in the nineteenth century—evolutionary biologists Charles Darwin and Thomas Henry Huxley. For Huxley, the death of his rambunctious son Noel came suddenly. They played before bedtime on a Thursday and Noel was dead by Saturday. It was for Huxley, as a friend wrote, "something horrible, intolerable, like being burnt alive." For Darwin, the death of his daughter Annie might be said to be worse, taking months as it did. Darwin, Gould writes, loved his frail little girl with a fierce tenderness. She had a sweet disposition and reminded Charles of his sister, who had helped raise him after their mother died early. Upon his daughter's death in April 1851, Darwin was devastated. "We can neither see on any side a gleam of comfort," he wrote. The dark feeling never entirely left him.

Too many children are dying needlessly around the world today, not for reasons beyond our comprehension, but because human attention was diverted and politics shifted a degree or two on the scale from public-spirited to self-driven. We may have lost the momentum we had built up through most of the twentieth century, but as Jon Mann reminded me, we must recognize how considerable our powers are to achieve progress, and that we do not need to rebuild the whole machine, far from it. There have been few such chances for humans in the long history of the race to achieve a dramatic turnaround, and rarely have they been so clear. But here we are; and we must choose. We will choose even if we do so by inaction.

There are few who will not acknowledge that our current world and its running globalization are scary. We can see the possibilities if it all works out, but we also know we've already made some mistakes. In such a time of confusion our best chance is to set aside our self-feeding emotions and our worldly cynicism and do the right thing, the bold stroke. It is not easy, but it's the best we've got. God help us if we continue to starve the system that supports us.

In fact, the picture now is not as bleak as the data suggest, because the work of recent years has drawn attention to the coming trouble.

Organizations like the Global Fund to Fight AIDS, Tuberculosis and Malaria have found clever and effective ways around the old patterns of slow and ineffectual aid. As we consider the urgency of generating full support for moving forward with this "new Marshall Plan," we would do well to consider two cautionary tales from the not too distant past.

Twice before the leading industrialized nations have found themselves confronting the challenges brought on by rapid globalization. After all, the first great globalization that rose up out of the nineteenth century crashed at the beginning of the twentieth when a terrorist act brought on World War I. Even after the long, grinding conflict, with new weapons and bloody casualties on a new scale, nations seemed unable to sit for long sessions of cooperation. An attempt to build a system of international trade and health organizations came to naught because the key nations could not, just as now, seem to agree on strategy. Cooperative trade and money exchange failed. The bubble of capitalist hopes was burst and a global economic depression ensued, accompanied by violent labor revolts. Soon a second great war followed.

The next time, however, the United States stepped forward to lead the building of an international cooperative system, even though its success seemed dubious. The United Nations was founded in San

Francisco and headquartered in New York. Europe, after several years and hundreds of millions of dollars of aid, was failing to regain its feet, and it appeared possible that Europe was sliding toward a permanent state like that we now see in developing countries. Some American leaders understood the problem and soon put forward the Marshall Plan. It was controversial because it sent huge sums of American money—with no guarantees—to countries that were sliding backward. There was worry that it would be stolen or misspent. The plan was also resisted as hopelessly idealistic, not to mention far too costly for an American nation just out of war. Some also wanted to direct America's attention more directly against the threat of the rising Soviet Union rather than take the "indirect" approach of building up the economies of our allies. But the Marshall Plan investment, which in today's dollars would have amounted to $100 billion to $200 billion over four years, turned out to be brilliant. So brilliant, in fact, that revisionist historians have said it was really a plot from the beginning by the United States to create and dominate a European market. The Europeans, however, are not complaining.

We have come again to a time when the world's economic powerhouses can promise decades of progress if they can work together. The groups and individuals who have rallied around the Millennium Development Project goals and the initiatives of the Global Fund to Fight AIDS, Tuberculosis and Malaria seem to be pulling in generally the same direction, and with a generally high belief that major progress around the world is possible. Or perhaps, that major progress is necessary if we don't want to see disease outbreaks and social and political unrest like those that characterized the end of the first great globalization.

Experts argue that the greater the participation of the United States, the greater the chance of building momentum quickly. The United States has been engaged—some would say mired—in a campaign to extend democracy around the world in the wake of the rise of global terrorism. Those efforts must now be complemented by an equally energetic push to spread good health to all corners of our troubled world.

The question of whether or not it is prudent to hope for such progress is answered, I think, by one recent story from New York. The poet Louis Simpson lives near a small beach and harbor on Long Island. For two months in the summer it is infested with vacationers, and the air is filled with the earsplitting racket of motorboats and water scooters. "The beach is littered with seat cushions, plastic containers, bottles . . . anything that can fall or be thrown from a boat," he wrote.

Each evening the poet and his wife walk on the beach, and each evening they bring a bag and pick up broken glass. When they began to do this, they realized it was futile. "We would never be able to pick up all the glass," he wrote.

But oddly enough, they *did* clean the harbor beach themselves, "for we take this walk every day if it isn't actually raining or snowing."

In this little story the will to address an intractable problem came first. Only later did it become clear that the task could actually be accomplished. This kind of thing happens more often than we think in human affairs.

NOTES

p. 19 *"Over the past two decades the [public health] infrastructure has greatly deteriorated"* Senator Bill Frist, "Public Health and National Security: The Critical Role of Increased Federal Support," *Health Affairs,* November–December 2002.

p. 29 *"Human beings have gained an unprecedented degree of control over their environment"* Robert William Fogel, *The Escape from Hunger and Premature Death, 1700–2100: Europe, America, and the Third World* (Cambridge, UK: Cambridge University Press, 2004).

p. 30 *Health is the crowning achievement of modern humankind* James C. Riley, *Rising Life Expectancy: A Global History* (Cambridge, UK: Cambridge University Press, 2001).

p. 33 *Health "for all" could be achieved* Declaration of the International Conference on Primary Health Care, sponsored by the World Health Organization at Alma-ata, Kazakhstan, 1978.

p. 33 *"We spend vast sums to lengthen the lives of terminally ill patients"* Ronald J. Glasser, "We Are Not Immune," *Harper's Magazine,* October 2004.

p. 45 *For Fazle Abed, it was the end of one life, the start of another* Personal interview, 2004.

p. 65 *Bill Gates Sr. once visited a BRAC village school* Speech by Bill Gates Sr. at the Global Health Council meeting in Washington, D.C., 2004.

p. 77 *It was eventually called "vitamania"* Scott Shane, Series of articles in the *Baltimore Sun*, October 2000.

p. 79 *This time, the reaction when the study was published was not silence* Personal interview with Alfred Sommer, 2004.

p. 84 *Shrestha is the fourth of seven children born in a farming village* Personal interview with Ram Shrestha, 2004.

p. 106 *"Well, by the grace of God, our child is in good health."* Quoted from a household discussion in Muzzafarnagar, India, October 2004.

p. 113 *"When you have a vaccine and deliver it to a household"* Personal interview with Dr. David Heymann in Moradabad, India, October 2004.

p. 138 *Gradually, Merck executives and Harvard public health doctors were learning* Personal interviews with Merck executives, including Guy MacDonald, 2002.

p. 152 *"This was not the way to run a national emergency"* Personal interview with Ernest Darkoh, 2002.

p. 155 *When he arrived back from his training in the United States* Personal interview with Ndwapi Ndwapi, 2003.

p. 172 *"Once it had arrived," wrote historian Richard J. Evans* Richard J. Evans, *Death in Hamburg: Society and Politics in the Cholera Years, 1830–1910* (London: Penguin Books, 1987).

p. 186 *"By the late 1970s, I had concluded that for all the good intentions and abilities"* Martin Wolf, *Why Globalization Works* (New Haven: Yale University Press, 2004).

p. 191 *"A revolution in economic thinking has taken place"* David Bloom and David Canning, "Health and Wealth of Nations," *Science,* February 2004.

p. 195 *Richard Feachem, one of the contributors to the report, explained, "The question became how can you buy the most dallies for your dollar?"* Richard Feachem, personal interview, 2004.

p. 199 *In the new world order "turmoil and chaos are increasingly emanating from undefined sources"* Jennifer Brower and Peter Chalk, *The Global Threat of New and Emerging Infectious Diseases: Reconciling U.S. National Security and Public Health Policy* (Santa Monica: Rand Corporation, 2003), 33.

p. 200 *"It is an alternative way of seeing the world"* Lloyd Axeworthy, quoted in Brower and Chalk, *Global Threat.* Ramesh Thakur is also quoted from the same source.

p. 206 *"The point is that with the Global Fund, it is all time-bound."* The Global Fund to Fight AIDS, Tuberculosis and Malaria annual report, 2004.

p. 206 *Aid for Africa in 2002, for example, amounted to a total of $30 per person* Jeffrey D. Sachs, *The End of Poverty: Economic Possibilities for Our Time* (New York: The Penguin Press, 2005).

p. 211 *People had dropped the old view of "Africa as an impossible continent"* Richard Horton, *Health Wars: On the Global Frontlines of Modern Medicine* (New York: New York Review Books, 2003).

p. 213 *"We say we are a free-trade society"* Bob Geldof, quoted from his presentation at the Commission on Africa, March 11, 2005.

p. 220 *"The Soviets were doing everything possible to achieve a complete breakdown of Europe."* Ed Cray, *General of the Army: George C. Marshall, Soldier and Statesman* (New York: Cooper Square Press, 2000).

p. 220 *So it was on that Tuesday after Marshall returned from Moscow* David McCullough, *Truman* (New York: Simon & Schuster, 1992).

p. 221 *"A rebellious House of Representatives"* Cray, *General of the Army.*

p. 222 *Allen Dulles, writing about the different approach of the Marshall plan* Allen Dulles, *The Marshall Plan* (Providence, RI: Berg Publishers, 1993).

p. 222 *It put the aid morally above all contention* Willy Brandt, former West German Chancellor, from a speech at Harvard University on the twenty-fifth anniversary of the Marshall Plan.

p. 224 *"It is not a philanthropic enterprise"* Dulles, *The Marshall Plan.*

p. 224 *"We need markets—big markets—in which to buy and sell"* Cray, *General of the Army.*

p. 225 *"Critics say dollars will not save Europe"* Dulles, *The Marshall Plan.*

p. 227 *It was built in the United States in a bipartisan fashion and it worked multi-laterally* W.W. Rostow, *The Stages of Economic Growth: A Non-Communist Manifesto* (Cambridge UK: Cambridge University Press, 1960).

SELECT BIBLIOGRAPHY

Bhagwati, Jagdish. *In Defense of Globalization*. New York: Oxford University Press, 2004.

Brower, Jennifer, and Peter Chalk. *The Global Threat of New and Reemerging Infectious Diseases: Reconciling U.S. National Security and Public Health Policy*. Santa Monica: Rand Corporation, 2003.

Commission on Macroeconomics and Health. *Macroeconomics and Health: Investing in Health for Economic Development*. Final report of the commission, 2001.

Easterly, William. *The Elusive Quest for Growth: Economists' Adventures and Misadventures in the Tropics*. Cambridge, MA: The MIT Press, 2002.

Fogel, Robert William. *The Escape from Hunger and Premature Death, 1700–2100: Europe, America, and the Third World*. Cambridge, UK: Cambridge University Press, 2004.

Horton, Richard. *Health Wars: On the Global Frontlines of Modern Medicine*. New York: New York Review Books, 2003.

James, Harold. *The End of Globalization: Lessons from the Great Depression.* Cambridge, MA: Harvard University Press, 2001.

Jamison, Dean, et al., editors. *Investing in Health: The World Development Report 1993.* Oxford: Oxford University Press, 1993.

Kim, Jim Yong, et al., editors. *Dying for Growth: Global Inequality and the Health of the Poor.* Monroe, ME: Common Courage Press, 2000.

Levine, Ruth. *Millions Saved: Proven Successes in Global Health.* Washington, D.C.: Center for Global Development, 2004.

Markel, Howard. *When Germs Travel: Six Major Epidemics that Have Invaded America Since 1900 and the Fears They Have Unleashed.* New York: Pantheon Books, 2004.

National Academy of Sciences, Institute of Medicine. *America's Vital Interest in Global Health: Protecting Our People, Enhancing Our Economy, and Advancing Our International Interests.* Washington, D.C.: National Academies Press, 1997.

———. *Emerging Infections: Microbial Threats to Health in the United States.* Washington, D.C.: National Academies Press, 1992.

———. *The Future of Public Health.* Washington, D.C.: National Academies Press, 1988.

———. *The Future of the Public's Health in the Twenty-First Century.* Washington, D.C.: National Academies Press, 2002.

———. *The Threat of Pandemic Influenza: Are We Ready?* Washington, D.C.: National Academies Press, 2005.

Riley, James C. *Rising Life Expectancy: A Global History.* Cambridge, UK: Cambridge University Press, 2001.

Sachs, Jeffrey D. *The End of Poverty: Economic Possibilities for Our Time.* New York: The Penguin Press, 2005.

Soros, George. *George Soros on Globalization.* New York: Public Affairs, 2002.

Stiglitz, Joseph E. *Globalization and its Discontents.* New York: W.W. Norton & Company, 2003.

Wolf, Martin. *Why Globalization Works.* New Haven: Yale University Press, 2004.

Resources

There are many opportunities to work on global health, from further reading and volunteer work in the United States to volunteer work in countries around the world and even "volunteer vacations" in many nations. The following guide to information, organizations, and volunteering will give readers a start.

GLOBAL HEALTH NEWS AND INFORMATION

Because news organizations in general have very poor and limited coverage of global health issues, it is necessary to seek out specialized sites and publications. Here are a few of the best.

HARVARD'S GLOBAL HEALTH NEWS
www.worldhealthnews.harvard.edu
An excellent site with stories selected from a great variety of publications each week.

KAISER FAMILY FOUNDATION'S GLOBAL HEALTH REPORTING
www.globalhealthreporting.org
A new site funded by the Bill and Melinda Gates Foundation. It gives regularly updated news and information on AIDS, malaria, and tuberculosis around the world. It includes tools for journalists, basic definitions, and lists of internships and other opportunities.

HEALTH E
www.health-e.org.za
Lots of news, and in-depth reporting by African journalists on HIV/AIDS and its politics as well as other public health issues in southern Africa, primarily South Africa.

AIDS EDUCATION GLOBAL INFORMATION SYSTEM (AEGIS)
www.aegis.com
A grassroots archive of worldwide AIDS information collected over the years and updated hourly.

ALL AFRICA
http://allafrica.com
A news source for stories from Africa, including many health stories from around the continent.

MAJOR ORGANIZATIONS

GLOBAL HEALTH COUNCIL
www.globalhealth.org
The largest membership organization on the subject, it comprises mainly professionals who work in health and development projects. The group uses only a few volunteers in its American offices, but its Web site offers a variety

of news and information about global health, including a regular newsletter with good, current reports.

Oxfam

www.oxfam.org

A large U.K. based charity that focuses on poverty and health issues. It accepts volunteers in its offices but doesn't send volunteers overseas. Their in-depth reports on world health issues are often very good.

Bill and Melinda Gates Foundation

www.gatesfoundation.org

A granting organization with an endowment of about $28 billion. Its Web site has a variety of useful information. It does not accept volunteers itself, but recommends volunteering in its grantee organizations.

Open Society Institute

www.soros.org

A grantmaking organization founded by George Soros that concentrates its work in Eastern Europe and the former Soviet Union. In addition to giving grants, it offers fellowships and scholarships.

Doctors Without Borders/Médecins Sans Frontières

In the U.S.: www.doctorswithoutborders.org

Internationally: www.msf.org

A worldwide professional and advocacy organization. The Web site offers articles on current activities and accepts volunteers.

Centers for Disease Control and Prevention

www.CDC.gov

Authoritative medical articles on many disease outbreaks from around the world.

WORLD HEALTH ORGANIZATION

www.who.int

A large, awkwardly-organized site with a lot of useful information.

PARTNERS IN HEALTH

www.pih.org

An organization largely for helping medical professionals carry out projects in other nations. The organization does ask for volunteers for advocacy work in the United States.

THE GLOBAL FUND TO FIGHT AIDS, TUBERCULOSIS AND MALARIA

www.theglobalfund.org

A grantmaking organization for global health that accepts donations not only from governments and NGOs, but from individuals as well.

THE UNITED NATIONS MILLENNIUM PROJECT

www.unmillenniumproject.org

The organization that is pressing nations to give more aid for poverty and health investments, and by agreement of UN members, has set out goals for development projects and their funding.

VOLUNTEER WORK

There are many volunteer opportunities available, from a wide variety of organizations. The first step in looking for such work is probably to look at overview sites and places where you may get advice on the first steps to volunteering. The Gates Organization has such advice at www.gatesfoundation.org; look under volunteering.

Several portal sites that contain thousands of volunteer listings are:

www.idealist.org
This includes many international volunteering program links.

www.volunteermatch.org
This site has volunteer links for thousands of jobs in the United States.

www.onesmallplanet.com
A site based at the University of Wisconsin that gives advice on volunteering and offers links to volunteer programs including "volunteer vacations," in which the volunteer pays to travel but works in a development program upon arrival.

www.volunteerinternational.org
The International Volunteer Programs Association is an alliance of nonprofit organizations based in the Americas that provide opportunities for volunteer work and internships.

These are specific links to some of the reputable and popular programs for international volunteering:

www.crossculturalsolutions.org
Cross-cultural Solutions

www.hvousa.org
Health Volunteers Overseas

www.globalvolunteers.org
Global Volunteer Network

www.amizade.org
Amizade

www.amigoslink.org
Amigos de las Americas

INDEX

social disruption and, 3

twentieth-century booms, 2

Elusive Quest for Growth, The (Easterly), 187–88

Emergency Plan for AIDS Relief, 37

encephalitis, 12–13

End of Poverty, The (Sachs), 214–15

Epidemic Intelligence Service, 73

Evans, Richard J., 172

Fantan, Tsetsele, 153

Farr, William, 178

FDA (Food and Drug Administration), 35

Feachem, Richard, 190, 195, 203, 206

Financial Times, 186

Fogel, Robert, 29–30, 195

Food and Drug Administration (FDA), 35

foreign aid, 43, 169

African statistics on, 206–7

to Asian Tigers, 72

debate about, to developing countries, 71–72, 183–89

history of, 26–27

myths about, 207–8

poverty in developing countries and, 200–202

renewed commitment to, need for, 210–15

vitamin A program as successful, 72

Foreign Policy, 185, 200–201

Foreign Service Journal, 71

Freedom House, 207

Friedman, Thomas, 3

Gandhi, Mahatma, 66

Gannon, John, 196

Garrett, Laurie, 6

Gates, Bill, 25

Gates, Bill Sr., 65

Gates Foundation, 139, 153

GDP (gross domestic product), as false measure of wealth, 194

Geldof, Bob, 213

Ghana, public health funding in, 205

Gilmartin, Ray, 139

Glasser, Ronald, 33–34

Global Fund to Fight AIDS, Tuberculosis and Malaria, 37, 167, 201, 203–6, 210, 211, 236, 237

global health. *See* public health

Global Health Council, 96

globalization, 2–6

diseases' evolution, effect on, 8–10

enlightened, 188, 190, 203, 215

nineteenth-century, 169

outbreak of disease during latest, 6–7

Global Program on Aids, 232

Global Vaccine Initiative, 26

Goldstone, Jack, 196

Gould, Stephen Jay, 234

government(s)

failure of national, 197–98

main duties of, 168

grandmothers of Nepal and vitamin A program, 91–94

gross domestic product (GDP) as false measure of wealth, 194

Gurr, Ted Robert, 196

hantavirus. *See* mad cow disease

Harvard AIDS Institute, 133, 138

Hazard, Ellen Isabella, 170–71, 181

health. *See* public health

Helms, Jessee, 26

comment on foreign aid and, 71

Heritage Foundation, 71

Heymann, David, 113, 162

H5N1. *See* avian flu

H6N2 flu, 17

Hong Kong flu, 16, 18

horizontal public health programs, 117–18, 204

Horton, Richard, 211

human capital, 190–91, 213

Huxley, Thomas Henry, 235

India, 38, 54, 229

Muslim workers in polio program in, 118–19

polio vaccine in, 104–7, 113–22, 125–29

Indian Council for Medical Research, 55

National Polio Surveillance Project, 113
national security
    factors affecting, 197–202
    human security vs., 200
Natsios, Andrew, 71, 136
Ndwapi, Ndwapi, 155–58
Nehru, Jawaharlal, 66
Nepal, 38, 81–83, 229
    grandmothers of, and vitamin A program, 91–94
    night blindness in, 68–70
    pneumonia program in, 97–100
    vitamin A program in, 84–95
Nepali National Vitamin A Program, 69
"new Marshall Plan," 25–26, 236
New York Times, 3
NGOs (non-governmental organizations), 46, 204, 231
Nigeria, outbreak of polio in, 121–25
night blindness
    in Nepal, 68–70
    as public health issue, 70–71
    research into causes of, 72–81
    science of, 73
    vitamin A program for, in Nepal, 84–95
    West Java study on, 73–75
non-governmental organizations (NGOs), 46, 204, 231
nutritional science, 76–77

Obasanjo, Olusegun, 210
oral rehydration therapy (ORT), 23
    costs of, in Bangladesh programs, 62
    creation of simple solutions of, 56–58
    as diarrhea treatment, 49–50
    early research in, 53–54
    misunderstanding of, by Bangladesh villagers, 59–61
outbreak(s)
    AIDS, 5–6, 12
    cholera, in nineteenth century as first global epidemic, 170–71
    cholera, in Peru, 14
    Ebola, 12
    encephalitis, 12–13

lassa fever, 12
Legionnaire's disease, 12
lyme disease, 12
Marburg fever, 5, 12
polio, 108–9, 121–25
public health system's effect on, 19–22
SARS (Severe Acute Respiratory Syndrome), 6, 11
West Nile disease, 12
Oxfam, 26

Panama Canal, 2
Pakistan-Bangladesh war, 44–45
Pfizer, 137
Philippines, 78–79
Phillips, Robert, 53
physical capital, 190–91
pneumonia, 22
    Nepalese program to combat, 97–100
polio, 229
    eradication of, as largest public health project, 103–4
    eradication of, in Bangladesh, 48
    history of outbreak of, 108–9
    Indian villagers' reluctance toward vaccine for, 113–15
    in Muslim areas of world, 14–15
    outbreak of, in Nigeria, 121–25
    reemergence of, in Indonesia, 5
    science of, 109–10
    vaccine, 31–32, 104–7, 110–11, 113–15, 125–29
political consequences of outbreak of disease, 19–22
Poor Law, 175
poverty and its impact on disease, 175–76
Powell, Colin, 200–201
"protease inhibitors," 134
public health
    AIDS as greatest challenge to, 130
    backslide in, since 1980s, 33–35
    budget for, 7, 15, 24, 35–36
    call for new initiatives in, 25–26
    community involvement in, in developing countries, 95–96

public health (*cont.*)
  curtailing night blindness and, 70–71
  deteriorating systems of, 19–22
  difficulty in executing, in developing countries,
    83–84
  economic progress and, 188–89
  foreign aid to developing countries and, 183–89
  as growth factor in economics, 191–95
  initiatives in current, 36–38
  life expectancy and, 28–29
  Millions Saved report on, 229–32
  Muslim mistrust of programs of, 121–25
  national security and, 198–202
  need for new initiatives in, 25–26
  during nineteenth-century cholera epidemic,
    172–73
  past improvements in, 27–28
  polio elimination as largest project in, 103–4
  sanitation's effect on, 30–31
  smallpox eradication and, 32
  successful programs, features of, 162–64
  vaccines' effect on, 31–32
  vertical and horizontal programs in, 117–18,
    204
Public Health Act, 168, 182

Radelet, Steven, 185, 200–201
Rand Corporation, 26, 196, 199
Riley, James, 29–30
Rohde, John, 56
Rostow, Walt Whitman, 183–85, 226–27
rotavirus, 49
Russia. *See* Soviet Union
Rwanda, 139

Sachs, Jeffrey, 24–25, 37, 188, 190, 195, 206, 214–15
Sahba, Naysan, 115–16, 118, 120–21, 128
"sanitarians," 31
sanitation
  public health and, 30–31
  in nineteenth-century London, 176–77, 180–82,
    216
Sarkar, Hemlata, 58
SARS (Severe Acute Respiratory Syndrome), 6, 11

Science, 191
Senate Foreign Relations Committee, 222, 223
Senegal, 139, 146
September 11, 2001, terrorist attacks, 15, 21
Severe Acute Respiratory Syndrome (SARS), 6, 11
sexual behavior
  comparison of Western and African, 142–43
  impact on transmission of AIDS, 143–46
Shane, Scott, 77
Sharma, Yamuna, 68–70
Shell Oil, 44
shigella, 49
Shrestha, Ram, 82, 84–95, 101–2, 162
Simpson, Louis, 238
Singh, Manmohan, 195
Singh, Sudeep Gadok, 112, 115–17, 120, 128–29
smallpox, 10, 103
  eradication of, 32, 107–8
Smith, Adam, 168, 174, 212, 213
Snow, John, 177–82
society, greatest achievements of, 30
Sommer, Alfred, 72–75, 78–79
South Africa, 23
Southward and Vauxhall Water Company, 178–79
Soviet Union, 199, 218, 220, 222, 227
Stages of Economic Growth, The (Rostow), 183
Stalin, Joseph, 219–20
"State Failure Task Force Report" (University of
    Maryland), 19–22
Stiglitz, Joseph, 188
Suez Canal, 2
Sunderland, England, 169
  quarantine of, 170–71
Swaziland, 23
syphilis, 10

Tagore, Rabindranath, 65
Taylor, Mary, 96
Teresa, Mother, 46
terrorism, 21–22
  poverty's link with, 201
  reaction to BRAC, 64–65
Thailand, 146
Thakur, Ramesh, 200

About the Author

Philip J. Hilts, the author of five books, has been a prize-winning health and science reporter for both *The New York Times* and *The Washington Post*. Over twenty years' time he placed more than three hundred stories on the front pages of those papers. His most recent book, *Protecting America's Health: The FDA, Business and 100 Years of Regulation* was named a *New York Times* Notable Book of the Year and the 2003 winner of the *Los Angeles Times* Book Prize for Science and Technology. Hilts has also taught science journalism to graduate students at Boston University and, more recently, taught journalism to undergraduates at the University of Botswana.